Molecular, Therapeutic, and Surgical Updates on Head and Neck Vascular Anomalies

Editors

SRINIVASA RAMA CHANDRA
SANJIV NAIR

ORAL AND MAXILLOFACIAL SURGERY CLINICS OF NORTH AMERICA

www.oralmaxsurgery.theclinics.com

Consulting Editor
RUI P. FERNANDES

February 2024 • Volume 36 • Number 1

ELSEVIER

1600 John F. Kennedy Boulevard • Suite 1800 • Philadelphia, Pennsylvania, 19103-2899

http://www.oralmaxsurgery.theclinics.com

ORAL AND MAXILLOFACIAL SURGERY CLINICS OF NORTH AMERICA Volume 36, Number 1
February 2024 ISSN 1042-3699, ISBN-13: 978-0-443-13015-1

Editor: John Vassallo; j.vassallo@elsevier.com
Developmental Editor: Anita Chamoli

Oral and Maxillofacial Surgery Clinics of North America (ISSN 1042-3699) is published quarterly by Elsevier Inc., 360 Park Avenue South, New York, NY 10010-1710. Months of issue are February, May, August, and November. Business and Editorial Offices: 1600 John F. Kennedy Blvd., Suite 1800, Philadelphia, PA 19103-2899. Periodicals postage paid at New York, NY and additional mailing offices. Subscription prices are $417.00 per year for US individuals, $100.00 per year for US students/residents, $488.00 per year for Canadian individuals, $100.00 per year for Canadian students/residents, $540.00 per year for international individuals, $235.00 per year for international students/residents. For institutional access pricing please contact Customer Service via the contact information below. To receive student/resident rate, orders must be accompanied by name or affiliated institution, date of term, and the *signature* of program/residency coordinator on institution letterhead. Orders will be billed at individual rate until proof of status is received. Foreign air speed delivery is included in all *Clinics* subscription prices. All prices are subject to change without notice. **POSTMASTER:** Send address changes to *Oral and Maxillofacial Surgery Clinics of North America,* Elsevier Periodicals **Customer Service, 11830 Westline Industrial Drive, St. Louis, MO 63146. Tel: 1-800-654-2452 (U.S. and Canada); 314-447-8871 (outside U.S. and Canada). Fax: 314-447-8029. E-mail: journalscustomerservice-usa@elsevier.com (for print support); journalsonlinesupport-usa@elsevier.com (for online support)**.

Reprints. For copies of 100 or more, of articles in this publication, please contact the Commercial Reprints Department, Elsevier Inc., 360 Park Avenue South, New York, NY 10010-1710. Tel.: 212-633-3874; Fax: 212-633-3820; Email: reprints@elsevier.com.

Oral and Maxillofacial Surgery Clinics of North America is covered in *MEDLINE/PubMed* (*Index Medicus*), *Science Citation Index Expanded (SciSearch®)*, *Journal Citation Reports/Science Edition*, and *Current Contents®/Clinical Medicine*.

Contributors

CONSULTING EDITOR

RUI P. FERNANDES, MD, DMD, FACS, FRCS(Ed)
Clinical Professor and Chief, Division of Head and Neck Surgery, Program Director, Head and Neck Oncologic Surgery and Microvascular Reconstruction Fellowship, Departments of Oral and Maxillofacial Surgery, Neurosurgery, and Orthopaedic Surgery and Rehabilitation, University of Florida Health Science Center, University of Florida College of Medicine, Jacksonville, Florida, USA

EDITORS

SRINIVASA RAMA CHANDRA, BDS, MD, FDS, FDSRCS(Eng), FIBCSOMS(Onc-Recon)
Associate Professor and Program Director, Department of Oral and Maxillofacial Surgery–Head and Neck Oncology and Microvascular Reconstruction, Oregon Health and Sciences University, Portland, Oregon, USA

SANJIV NAIR, MDS, FDS, FFD, FFDRCS, FDSRCPS, FIBSCOMS
Professor, Lead Clinician, Maxillofacial Surgery, Bhagwan Mahaveer Jain Hospital, Head, Bangalore Institute of Dental Sciences, Malleswaram, Bangalore, Karnataka, India

AUTHORS

ALLISON BRITT, MS, LCGC
Comprehensive Vascular Anomalies Program, Children's Hospital of Philadelphia, Philadelphia, Pennsylvania, USA

ANDREA B. BURKE, DMD, MD
Assistant Professor, Department of Oral and Maxillofacial Surgery, University of Washington School of Dentistry, Seattle, Washington, USA

ROSALÍA BALLONA CHAMBERGO, MD
Pediatric Dermatologist, Head of Dermatology, Instituto Nacional de Salud del Niño de Breña, Lima, Perú

SRINIVASA R. CHANDRA, BDS, MD, FDS, FDSRCS(Eng), FIBCSOMS (Onc-Recon)
Associate Professor and Program Director, Department of Oral and Maxillofacial

Surgery–Head and Neck Oncology and Microvascular Reconstruction, Oregon Health and Sciences University, Portland, Oregon, USA

CHAO DONG, MS
Predoctoral Student, University of Washington School of Dentistry, Seattle, Washington, USA

MADAN ETHUNANDAN, MDS, FRCS (OMFS), FDSRCS, FFDRCSI
Consultant Oral and Maxillofacial Surgeon, University Hospital Southampton, Southampton, United Kingdom; Visting Professor, Oral and Maxillofacial Surgery, Sri Ramachandra Institute of Higher Education and Research, Chennai, Tamil Nadu, India

LUCIANA DANIELA GARLISI TORALES, MD
Unit on Vascular Malformations, Division of Intramural Research, Eunice Kennedy Shriver National Institute for Child Health and Human Development, Bethesda, Maryland, USA

JORIE GATTS, MD
Clinical Fellow, Hemangioma and Vascular Malformation Center, Cancer and Blood Diseases Institute, Cincinnati Children's Hospital Medical Center, Cincinnati, Ohio, USA

JESSE G.A. JONES, MD
Assistant Professor of Radiology and Neurosurgery, The University of Alabama at Birmingham, Birmingham, Alabama, USA

ARSHAD KALEEM, DDS, MD
Associate Surgeon, El Paso Head and Neck and Microvascular Surgery, El Paso, Texas, USA

DEEPAK KRISHNAN, DDS, FACS
Associate Professor, Department of Surgery, Section of Oral and Maxillofacial Surgery, University of Cincinnati, University of Cincinnati College of Medicine, Cincinnati, Ohio, USA

BALASUBRAMANYA KUMAR, MDS, FIBCSOMS
Maxillofacial Surgeon, Maxillofacial Surgery, Bhagwan Mahaveer Jain Hospital, Bangalore, Karnataka, India

JAMES C. MELVILLE, DDS, FACS
Associate Professor, Bernard and Gloria Pepper Katz Department of Oral and Maxillofacial Surgery, Oral, Head and Neck Oncology and Microvascular Reconstructive Surgery, The University of Texas Health Science Center at Houston, Houston, Texas, USA

NADIA MEZGHANI, DDS
Resident PGY 1, Oral and Maxillofacial Surgery, Mount Sinai Health System and Jacobi Medical Center, Center, Bronx, New York, USA

ADVAITH NAIR
Department of Oral and Maxillofacial Surgery–Head and Neck Oncology and Microvascular Reconstruction, Oregon Health and Sciences University, Portland, Oregon, USA

SANJIV NAIR, MDS, FDS, FFD, FFDRCS, FDSRCPS, FIBSCOMS
Professor, Lead Clinician, Maxillofacial Surgery, Bhagwan Mahaveer Jain Hospital, Head, Bangalore Institute of Dental Sciences, Malleswaram, Bangalore, Karnataka, India

KAYLEE R. PURPURA, MD
Otolaryngologist, Department of Otolaryngology–Head and Neck Surgery, Oregon Health and Science University, Portland, Oregon, USA

RISHABH RATTAN, DDS
Resident PGY 1, Bernard and Gloria Pepper Katz Department of Oral and Maxillofacial Surgery, The University of Texas Health Science Center at Houston, Houston, Texas, USA

KIERSTEN RICCI, MD
Clinical Director, Hemangioma and Vascular Malformation Center, Assistant Professor of Pediatrics, Division of Hematology, Cancer and Blood Diseases Institute, Cincinnati Children's Hospital Medical Center, University of Cincinnati College of Medicine, Cincinnati, Ohio, USA

JOSHUA S. SCHINDLER, MD
Associate Professor, Department of Otolaryngology–Head and Neck Surgery, Oregon Health and Science University, Portland, Oregon, USA

ANJAN KUMAR SHAH, MDS, FDS, FFD, FIBCSOMS(Onco & Recon)
Maxillofacial Surgery, Bhagwan Mahaveer Jain Hospital, Oral and Maxillofacial Surgery, Rajarajeswari Dental College and Hospital, Bangalore, Karnataka, India

SARAH E. SHEPPARD, MD, PhD
Unit on Vascular Malformations, Division of Intramural Research, Eunice Kennedy Shriver National Institute for Child Health and Human Development, Bethesda, Maryland, USA

FELIPE VELASQUEZ VALDERRAMA, MD
Pediatric Dermatologist, Instituto Nacional de Salud del Niño de Breña, Lima, Perú

HELENA VIDAURRI DE LA CRUZ, MD
Pediatric Dermatologist, Dermato-Oncologist
and Dermatologic Surgeon, Pediatrician,
Department of Pediatrics, Hospital
General de México Dr. Eduardo Liceaga,
O.D. Health Ministry, Tenured Professor of
Dermatology, Faculty of Medicine, National
Autonomous University of Mexico, Mexico
City, Mexico

ALEJANDRO WOLF, DO
Department of Pathology, ARUP Laboratories,
University of Utah, Salt Lake City, Utah, USA

KRISTINA M. WOODIS, BS
Unit on Vascular Malformations, Division of
Intramural Research, Eunice Kennedy Shriver
National Institute for Child Health and Human
Development, Bethesda, Maryland, USA

Contents

Preface: Vascular Anomalies - Molecular, Testing and Management Updates　　　xi

Srinivasa Rama Chandra and Sanjiv Nair

Updates in Genetic Testing for Head and Neck Vascular Anomalies　　　1

Kristina M. Woodis, Luciana Daniela Garlisi Torales, Alejandro Wolf, Allison Britt, and Sarah E. Sheppard

> Vascular anomalies include benign or malignant tumors or benign malformations of the arteries, veins, capillaries, or lymphatic vasculature. The genetic etiology of the lesion is essential to define the lesion and can help navigate choice of therapy. . In the United States, about 1.2% of the population has a vascular anomaly, which may be underestimating the true prevalence as genetic testing for these conditions continues to evolve.

Lasers and Nonsurgical Modalities　　　19

Rishabh Rattan, Nadia Mezghani, Arshad Kaleem, and James C. Melville

> Head and neck vascular pathology is routinely encountered by the maxillofacial surgeon. Although these anomalies have been traditionally managed by surgical means, adjunctive therapies have been popularized in recent years. The use of laser therapy has gained attention for its ability to better access and to provide more predictable outcomes in the highly intricate and vascular areas of the head and neck. Laser therapy allows for the selective targeting of diseased tissue while maintaining the integrity of surrounding healthy tissue.

Indications, Options, and Updates on Embolic Agents　　　29

Jesse G.A. Jones

> Interventional approaches to head and neck vascular anomalies have evolved with our understanding of disease pathologic condition and advances in medical and surgical treatment. Embolization's role in the disease management ranges from standalone treatment with curative intent to adjunctive or even palliative, depending on the lesion. This decision is best made through multidisciplinary collaboration among surgeons, interventionalists, and medical specialists. Finally, setting realistic expectations with the patient and family is a crucial step preceding any intervention. This article elaborates on the considerations influencing a given treatment plan and specific interventional strategy.

Terminology and Classifications of Vascular Lesions Based on Molecular Identification　　　35

Srinivasa R. Chandra, Advaith Nair, and Sanjiv Nair

> The majority of the vascular anomalies are seen in the head and neck region. Even though the incidence of this anomaly could be construed as a rare disease entity, with only 5% of overall affliction, the lack of knowledgeable management has disfigured many. A comprehensive understanding of this benign yet complex life-changing entity is essential. A historical perspective, pathophysiology-logical evolution, and the current knowledge of management modalities are essential for rendering clinical care in this subspecialty care.

Dermatologic Review in Pediatric Vascular Lesions   49

Helena Vidaurri de la Cruz, Felipe Velasquez Valderrama, and Rosalía Ballona Chambergo

Vascular anomalies (VAs) can be present in any organ; however, the skin being the largest one, it is there where many of them are evident; some are visible at birth, others develop throughout life. Pediatric dermatologists are specially trained to distinguish VAs from their mimickers, which require different treatments and may harbor distinct prognoses. We resume the diagnostic and therapeutic tasks of pediatric dermatologist at our vascular anomaly clinics, as well as the differential diagnoses of mimickers of VAs.

Management of Midfacial and Skull Vault Osseous Vascular Lesions   61

Madan Ethunandan

There continuous to be widespread misuse of nomenclature used to described vascular anomalies, This is even more pronounced in the case of intra-osseous lesions. Bone involvement is more common with vascular malformations and extremely rare in haemangiomas. An accurate diagnosis is mandatory for tailored management and often based on a thorough history, clinical examination, and cross-sectional imaging. Surgery remains the main stay for the management of symptomatic venous malformations. Embolisation with or without surgery is the main stay for arteriovenous malformations. Virtual surgical planning, with surgical guides and patient specific implants help achieve predictably excellent results.

Airway Considerations in Vascular Lesions   73

Kaylee R. Purpura and Joshua S. Schindler

Vascular anomalies of the head and neck frequently involve the upper aerodigestive tract and can cause some level of airway obstruction. It is important to fully evaluate the extent of a lesion and resultant functional impairment with a flexible fiberoptic laryngoscopy. Treating these lesions is difficult and considering how to manage the airway during a procedure is critical. A multidisciplinary approach should be used for airway management with alternative intubation plans established prior to induction of anesthesia. Edema and hemorrhage are expected complications from the treatment of vascular anomalies and should be considered when planning for extubation at the end of a procedure.

Case Reviews in Head and Neck Vascular Lesion Management   81

Balasubramanya Kumar, Srinivasa R. Chandra, Sanjiv Nair, and Anjan Kumar Shah

The treatment of hemangiomas and vascular malformations should be individualized, based upon the size of the lesion(s), morphology, location, presence or possibility of complications, the potential for scarring or disfigurement, the age of the patient, and the rate of growth or involution at the time of evaluation. The major challenge is the location in a head and neck can lead to unsightly scars if approached improperly, or with inadequate approaches can lead to intraoperative and postoperative morbidity with neurovascular damage and inadequate lesion excision. Facial, trigeminal, and other cranial nerve branches are of key importance in the functional outcome while accessing and approaching head and neck vascular lesions.

Updates to the Management of Gorham–Stout Disease and Osseous Vascular Lesions in the Head and Neck   93

Andrea B. Burke, Chao Dong, and Srinivasa R. Chandra

Osseous vascular anomalies can be characterized as vascular tumors or malformations. Classification is vital for prognosis and treatment. Much remains unknown about conditions such as Gorham–Stout disease. Treatments target the proposed genetic pathways such as PI3KCA/AKT/mTOR pathway.

Medical Management of Nonmalignant Vascular Tumors of the Head and Neck: Part 1   **103**

Jorie Gatts, Srinivasa Chandra, Deepak Krishnan, and Kiersten Ricci

Vascular anomalies, broadly classified as nonmalignant tumors and malformations, consist of a multitude of disorders that have a wide range of symptoms and complications as well as overlapping clinical, radiologic, and histologic findings. Although usually difficult, distinguishing between nonmalignant vascular tumors and malformations, as well as the precise diagnosis within these distinctions, is critical because prognosis, therapy, and chronicity of care vary greatly. In contrast to normal endothelial turnover in vascular malformations, vascular tumors are characterized by the abnormal proliferation of endothelial cells and aberrant blood vessels.

Medical Management and Therapeutic Updates on Vascular Anomalies of the Head and Neck: Part 2   **115**

Jorie Gatts, Srinivasa R. Chandra, and Kiersten Ricci

Discovery of inherited and somatic genetic mutations, along with advancements in clinical and scientific research, has improved understanding of vascular anomalies and changed the treatment paradigm. With aim of minimizing need for invasive procedures and improving disease outcomes, molecularly targeted medications and anti-angiogenesis agents have become important as both adjuncts to surgery, and increasingly, as the primary treatment of vascular anomalies. This article highlights the commonly used and emerging therapeutic medications for non-malignant vascular tumors and vascular malformations in addition to medical management of associated hematologic abnormalities.

Medical Therapeutics for the Treatment of Vascular Anomalies: Part 3   **125**

Kiersten Ricci

The discovery of inherited and somatic genetic mutations, along with advancements in clinical and scientific research, has improved the understanding of vascular anomalies and changed the treatment paradigm. With the aim of minimizing the need for invasive procedures and improving disease outcomes, molecularly targeted medications and anti-angiogenesis agents have become important as both adjuncts to surgery, and increasingly, as the primary treatment of vascular anomalies. This article highlights the commonly used and emerging therapeutic medications for nonmalignant vascular tumors and vascular malformations.

ORAL AND MAXILLOFACIAL SURGERY CLINICS OF NORTH AMERICA

FORTHCOMING ISSUES

May 2024
Gender Affirming Surgery
Russell E. Ettinger, *Editor*

August 2024
Pediatric Craniomaxillofacial Pathology
Srinivas M. Susarla, *Editor*

November 2024
Perforator Flaps
Susana Heredero, *Editor*

RECENT ISSUES

November 2023
Pediatric Craniomaxillofacial Trauma
Srinivas M. Susarla, *Editor*

August 2023
Imaging of Common Oral Cavity, Sinonasal, and Skull Base Pathology
Dinesh Rao, *Editor*

May 2023
Diagnosis and Management of Oral Mucosal Lesions
Donald Cohen and Indraneel Bhattacharyya, *Editors*

SERIES OF RELATED INTEREST

Atlas of the Oral and Maxillofacial Surgery Clinics
www.oralmaxsurgeryatlas.theclinics.com

Dental Clinics
www.dental.theclinics.com

THE CLINICS ARE NOW AVAILABLE ONLINE!
Access your subscription at:
www.theclinics.com

Preface
Vascular Anomalies - Molecular, Testing and Management Updates

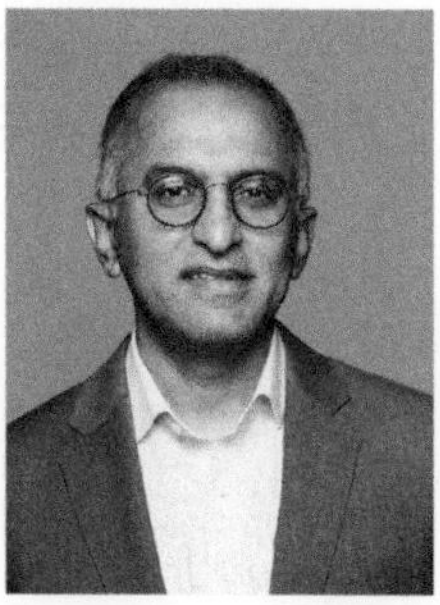

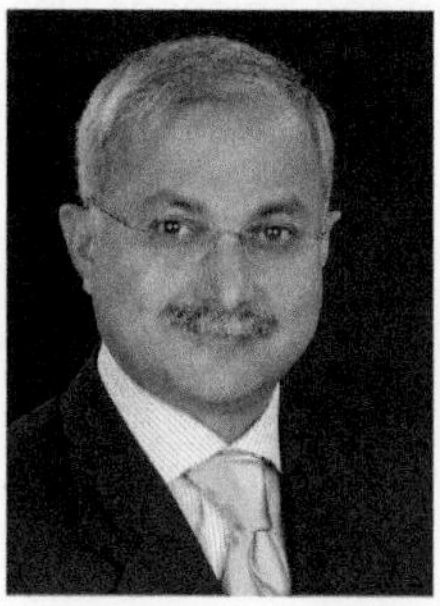

Srinivasa Rama Chandra, MD, BDS, FDSRCS(Eng), FIBCSOMS(Onc-Recon)   Sanjiv Nair, MDS, FFDRCS, FDSRCPS, FIBSCOMS
Editors

We thank each individual person and their families that we have encountered with vascular anomalies, their trust in our ability, the peers and authors who helped contribute to this endeavor, and our publishing team. We have done similar issues before, and there is lot more to do in helping to understand vascular anamolies. We hope you will read, learn, and teach us and provide care for many.

The first documented surgical exercise under a general anesthetic was a venous malformation of the head and neck. The philosophy of management and protocols has evolved ever since. Vascular anomalies present a plethora of clinical appearances and biological behaviors, making it an extremely clinical challenge to manage.

The understanding of their pathogenesis was a revelation, allowing diagnostic modalities and therapy. As imaging is the mainstay in the identification of this pathologic condition, there are modern images that identify the depth and extent of the lesion and the dynamics of blood flow.

Conventional management involves medical, surgical, and a combination of both. Use of interventional endovascular embolization provides safe ablation of these lesions.

Future management of these anomalies requires understanding of the angiogenesis of the blood vessels and the genetic mutations that lead to their formation.

Surgical advances create little morbidity with better aesthetic outcome. Use of navigational, endovascular interventions, and robotic access minimize blood loss intraoperatively. Reconstructive options with careful planning also provide better outcome with regenerative biomaterial use.

The future of vascular lesions and anomaly management rely on accurate classification and ontologically precise conceptual data. Mutations and pathway identification of each anomaly will lead to proliferative potential mechanism-targeted biological therapy. Further understanding of long-term outcomes of novel drug therapies based on the mammalian target of rapamycin (mTOR) and others will be evident to guide further trials.

We attribute William Osler's and Charles Darwin's advice of "observing the natural history" and "bedside medicine" in tandem. That is, not substituting for only technology or machine learning but use both of these to promote better understanding of molecular pathways. In addition, Osler's and Darwin's approach to disease as a unique condition in every individual and as not the same even if they morphologically appear to be "alike and behave similarly", leads to a future of only or maintained targeted medical therapy rather than mutilating surgery alone.

To all the future therapists and individuals affected with vascular anomalies, not "patients" or "doctors," we belive the horizon is bright! Please term the "anomaly" accurately and treat it *just adequately*. And as a footnote: vascular anomaly

Oral Maxillofacial Surg Clin N Am 36 (2024) xi–xii
https://doi.org/10.1016/j.coms.2023.09.009
1042-3699/24/© 2023 Published by Elsevier Inc.

treatment does not belong to a specialty but to an empathetic specialist—a person.

Srinivasa Rama Chandra, BDS,MD,
FDSRCS(Eng), FIBCSOMS(Onc-Recon)
Department of Oral and Maxillofacial Surgery–
Head and Neck Oncology and
Microvascular Reconstruction
Oregon Health and Sciences University
3181 SW Sam Jackson Park Road
Portland, OR 97239, USA

Sanjiv Nair, MDS, FFDRCS, FDSRCPS,
FIBSCOMS
B M Jain Hospital
Bangalore Institute of Dental Sciences
35, 4th Main 13 Cross
Malleswaram, Bangalore 560003, India

E-mail addresses:
chandrsr@ohsu.edu (S.R. Chandra)
snmaxfax@gmail.com (S. Nair)

*Corresponding author.

Updates in Genetic Testing for Head and Neck Vascular Anomalies

Kristina M. Woodis, BS[a], Luciana Daniela Garlisi Torales, MD[a],
Alejandro Wolf, DO[b], Allison Britt, MS, LCGC[c], Sarah E. Sheppard, MD, PhD[a],*

KEYWORDS

- Vascular malformation • Vascular anomaly • Genetics • PI3K signaling • RAS-MAPK signaling
- Somatic mosaicism

KEY POINTS

- Considerations for genetic testing include type of DNA, sample type, and breadth and depth of coverage.
- Slow-flow lesions are more likely to be caused by genes in the PI3K signaling pathway.
- Fast-flow lesions are more likely to be caused by genes in the RAS-MAPK signaling pathway.

INTRODUCTION

Vascular anomalies include benign or malignant vascular tumors or benign malformations of the arteries, veins, capillaries, or lymphatic vasculature. In the United States, about 1.2% of the population has a vascular anomaly.[1] Individuals with vascular anomalies may have chronic pain, recurrent infections, bleeding, clotting disorders, functional limitations, physical deformities, and poor quality of life. While some may resolve spontaneously, other vascular anomalies can severely decrease quality of life in patients if left untreated and may become life-threatening. Vascular anomalies are classified by the International Society for the Study of Vascular Anomalies.[2] In this review, the authors highlight both vascular tumors and vascular malformations of the head and neck. Vascular malformations may be classified by their vessel type. Accordingly, fast-flow vascular malformations refer to arteriovenous malformations where arteries shunt into veins, and slow-flow vascular malformations refer to malformations formed by dilated venous or lymphatic vessels.[3] Capillary malformations are the dilation of capillaries in large patches or telangiectasias, which are smaller malformations.[4] Additionally, the lymphatic vasculature may develop abnormally which can lead to cystic lymphatic malformations, leading to small or large pockets of dilated lymphatics, lymphedema, the accumulation of lymphatic fluid, or complex lymphatic anomalies, which involve lymphatic malformations affecting multiple organ systems.[5]

There are distinct molecular mechanisms that govern vascular development. Tyrosine kinase receptors, the phosphoinositide-3-kinase (PI3K) and the Rat sarcoma (RAS)-mitogen activated protein kinase (MAPK) pathways are essential components that direct growth and differentiation of endothelial cells (**Fig. 1**). Other signaling molecules define vessel identity, stability, and remodeling. Pathogenic variants (previously known as "mutations") in these genes result in a variety of vascular malformations. Identifying the genetic cause can direct medical screening and medical therapy,

[a] Unit on Vascular Malformations, Division of Intramural Research, *Eunice Kennedy Shriver* National Institute for Child Health and Human Development, 10 Center Drive, MSC 1103, Bethesda, MD 20892-1103, USA; [b] Department of Pathology and ARUP Laboratories, University of Utah, 2000 Circle of Hope, Room 3100, Salt Lake City, UT 84112, USA; [c] Comprehensive Vascular Anomalies Program, Children's Hospital of Philadelphia, Philadelphia, PA, USA
* Corresponding author. 10 Center Drive, MSC 1103, Bethesda, MD 20892-1103.
E-mail address: sarah.sheppard@nih.gov

Oral Maxillofacial Surg Clin N Am 36 (2024) 1–17
https://doi.org/10.1016/j.coms.2023.09.001

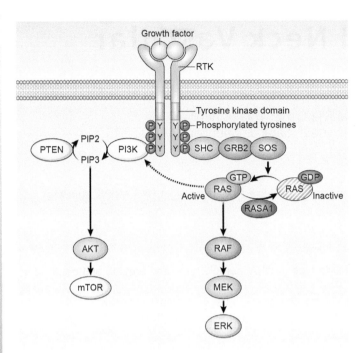

Fig. 1. Pathogenic variants in receptor tyrosine kinases, components of PI3K signaling, and components of RAS-MAPK signaling are important drivers of vascular anomalies.

provide information about prognosis and recurrence risk for other family members, and reassure family members about the exact cause of the anomaly.

The main objective of this review is to define the current known genetic causes of vascular anomalies of the head and neck. To accomplish this, the authors also address relevant topics such as inheritance, a limited review of genetic testing methods, and the molecularly targeted therapies currently in use.

Inheritance Patterns

Vascular anomalies may occur due to a pathogenic variant, a change in a gene that causes a disease phenotype, which can be inherited from family members via autosomal dominant inheritance or autosomal recessive inheritance. In other instances, patients may develop a vascular anomaly due to a pathogenic variant that developed after fertilization in some of their cells, known as somatic mosaicism.

Autosomal Dominant Inheritance

In autosomal dominant inheritance, an individual only needs one pathogenic variant on an allele to display the disease phenotype (**Fig. 2**A). Thus, autosomal dominant variants may be passed on to the next generation if a child receives the allele with the pathogenic variant from an affected

parent. In this type of inheritance, all individuals with a pathogenic variant are affected and there are no carriers. There is a 50% risk of recurrence.

Autosomal Recessive Inheritance

Like autosomal dominant inheritance, pathogenic variants may be passed on to next generations and appear in all cells. However, in autosomal recessive inheritance, two pathogenic variants in trans, one from each parent, are required to develop a disease phenotype (**Fig. 2**B). Thus, parents have the chance of having unaffected children, who did not receive any pathogenic variants, carrier children who have one copy of the pathogenic variant, or affected children who have two copies of the pathogenic variant: one inherited from each parent.

Somatic Mosaicism

Unlike autosomal inheritance, in which pathogenic variants are passed down to offspring through affected germline cells, a pathogenic variant may occur in somatic cells of the body during DNA replication after the zygote was formed, rather than in germline cells that lead to inheritance[6] (**Fig. 2**C). When individuals develop a phenotype in only a portion of their cells, rather than all cells, the pathogenic variant is classified as mosaic.[6] Therefore, a genetic test may only detect the pathogenic variant if it is taken from an area of affected

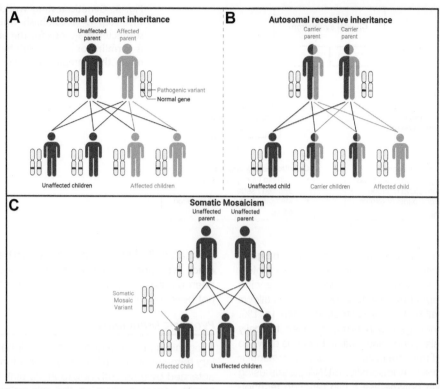

Fig. 2. Inheritance patterns. (*A*) Autosomal dominant inheritance. (*B*) Autosomal recessive inheritance. (*C*) Somatic mosaicism. Created with Biorender.

cells. This may complicate genetic testing if the affected site cannot be sampled or remains undetected.

GENETIC TESTING

Selecting the appropriate genetic test for a vascular anomaly requires 2 main considerations: the sample type(s) and the breadth and depth of coverage needed (**Fig. 3**, **Table 1**). It is helpful first to establish whether the clinician suspects a germline or a mosaic cause.

Sample type considerations include the type of DNA and the type of tissue. Currently, commercial genetic testing laboratories perform genetic testing on genomic DNA, or the DNA that is inside the nucleus of cells. Research has successfully shown that cell-free DNA (cfDNA), the DNA that is free-floating in biological fluids, isolated from blood or lymphatic cyst fluid is an adequate sample type for pathogenic variant detection.[7,8–12] Clinical genetic testing from cfDNA recently became available from blood or lymphatic fluid.[13] The other consideration is the type of tissue. In cases of mosaicism, a tissue sample of the vascular anomaly or "affected" tissue sample is needed. Some genetic testing laboratories will

pair testing with an "unaffected" tissue sample such as leukocyte DNA isolated from a saliva or blood sample for genetic comparison. The DNA quality is best when extracted from fresh or frozen tissue samples but newer technology has resulted in improved yields with formalin-fixed paraffin-embedded tissue.[14]

Both the breadth (number of genes) and depth (how many times an area of the genome is sequenced) are important in selecting the type of genetic test. Due to technical sequencing capabilities, tests with greater breadth may often have lower depth of coverage. In general, many panels for germline conditions will have sequencing coverage depth of approximately 30 to 50 × and tend to sequence the protein-coding regions of genes or the "exome" and then analyze a subset of genes. Exome sequencing evaluates the protein-coding regions of genes and genome sequencing will sequence the entire genome. Most genetic testing laboratories will include copy number variant detection with exome or genome sequencing.

Typically, gene panels, exomes, and genomes will not detect low-level mosaic variants or low variant allele fractions (the fraction of reads carrying the mosaic variant compared to the reference

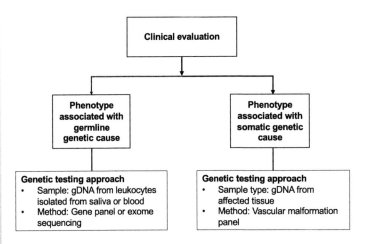

Fig. 3. Genetic testing workflow. The first step is to establish whether the suspected diagnosis for the phenotype is germline or mosaic. This helps determine the sample type and test to select.

sequence). In contrast, vascular malformation gene panels will initially capture specific regions of interest before sequencing, leading to sequencing coverage depth from 500 to 2000 $\times$.[15] This allows for variant allele fraction detection down to 1%. Although cancer gene panels may be used, typically cancer panels report variant allele fractions down to only 5% and may not include all genes for vascular malformations.[16] Additionally, cfDNA panels using digital droplet polymerase chain reaction technology will allow for detection of variant allele fractions below 1%.

VASCULAR TUMORS
Infantile Hemangioma

Infantile hemangiomas are the most common pediatric vascular tumors, occurring in about 4% of infants.[18] Risk factors for infantile hemangiomas include multiple gestation, prematurity, low birth weight, White race, female sex, and progesterone therapy, and family history.[17] Infantile hemangiomas are not present at birth, but will undergo a proliferative phase of growth (usually from about 3–12 months of age) followed by an involution stage that can last up to almost 10 years. Infantile hemangiomas are GLUT-1 positive by immunostaining, but currently no specific genetic cause has been identified.

Posterior Fossa Anomalies, Hemangioma, Arterial Anomalies, Cardiac Anomalies, and Eye Anomalies Association

Posterior fossa anomalies, hemangioma, arterial anomalies, cardiac anomalies, and eye anomalies (PHACE) association is the association of segmental infantile hemangiomas of the face with additional findings including posterior fossa abnormalities, arterial anomalies, cardiac malformations (including aortic coarctation), and eye

anomalies.[19–22] Sternal raphe may also be considered. Although extensive genetic research has been performed, a conclusive genetic cause has not been identified.[23]

Pyogenic Granuloma

Pyogenic granuloma, also known as lobular capillary hemangioma, is a benign vascular tumor characterized by a smooth or exophytic pink to red to purple papule present on the skin or mucosa.[24] Typically, histology will show lobular proliferations of capillaries (**Fig. 4**). Somatic pathogenic variants in RAS-MAPK genes including *NRAS, HRAS, KRAS, BRAF*, and *MAP2K1* likely resulting in activation of the RAS-MAPK pathway have been found in pyogenic granulomas, though *BRAF c.1799T>A* appears to be the most common driver pathogenic variant.[24–26]

Tufted Angioma and Kaposiform Hemangioendothelioma

Tufted angioma (TA) is a benign, childhood, vascular tumor that is typically stable or may regress spontaneously. The genetic cause for TA is also not well established. *NRAS* p.Q61R and *GNA14* were found in tissue from a single individual with TA.[27,28] Notably, tufted angioma and Kaposiform hemangioendothelioma (KHE) are thought to be related as they have similar methylation profiles.[28] KHE is a rare, benign vascular tumor that typically presents with reddish-purplish skin lesions with poorly-defined borders.[30] The genetic cause of KHE is poorly defined—a *RAD50* variant was identified in one KHE sample and *GNA14* was identified in one sample.[27,28]

FAST-FLOW VASCULAR MALFORMATIONS

Fast-Flow vascular malformations are those involving arteries which have fast flow. These are

Table 1
Phenotype-genotype associations for vascular malformations

Phenotype	Genotype	Inheritance	Genetic Testing Options
Infantile hemangioma	N/A		
Posterior fossa malformations, hemangioma, arterial anomalies, coarctation of the aorta/cardiac defects, and eye abnormalities (PHACE) association	N/A		
Pyogenic granuloma	NRAS, HRAS, KRAS, BRAF, and MAP2K1	Somatic mosaicism	Deep vascular gene panel
Tufted angioma	*Single cases reported with NRAS, GNA14	Somatic mosaicism	Deep vascular gene panel
Kaposiform hemangioendothelioma	*Single cases reported with RAD50, GNA14	Somatic mosaicism	Deep vascular gene panel
Sporadic arteriovenous malformations	KRAS, BRAF, MAP2K1, HRAS	Somatic mosaicism	Deep vascular gene panel
Capillary malformation arteriovenous malformation syndrome (CM-AVM)	RASA1 EPHB4	Autosomal dominant	Germline vascular panel; consider whether to include HHT genes
Hereditary hemorrhagic telangiectasia (HHT)	ENG, ACVRL1, SMAD4, and GDF2	Autosomal dominant	Germline vascular panel; consider whether to include CM-AVM genes
PTEN hamartoma of soft tissue	PTEN	Autosomal dominant or Somatic mosaicism	Deep vascular gene panel including PTEN or PTEN germline testing depending on the phenotype
Mucocutaneous venous malformation	TEK	Autosomal dominant	Germline vascular panel; consider whether deep vascular gene panel would be helpful or if it would be helpful to include GLMN
Sporadic venous malformation	TEK PIK3CA (less common)	Somatic mosaicism	Deep vascular gene panel
Blue rubber bleb nevus syndrome	TEK	Somatic mosaicism	Deep vascular gene panel
Cystic lymphatic malformation	PIK3CA BRAF, PIK3R1, KRAS (less common)	Somatic mosaicism	Deep vascular gene panel
Mixed slow-flow malformation	PIK3CA	Somatic mosaicism	Deep vascular gene panel

(continued on next page)

Table 1
(continued)

Phenotype	Genotype	Inheritance	Genetic Testing Options
Glomuvenous malformation	GLMN	Autosomal dominant	Germline vascular panel; consider whether deep vascular gene panel would be helpful or if it would be helpful to include TEK
Verrucous venous malformation	MAPK3K3	Somatic mosaicism	Deep vascular gene panel
Familial cerebral cavernous malformation (CCM)	CCM1 (KRIT1), CCM2 (MGC4607), or CCM3 (PDCD10)	Autosomal dominant	Germline CCM gene panel; consider whether deep vascular gene panel would be helpful
Sporadic cerebral cavernous malformation	CCM1 (KRIT1), CCM2 (MGC4607), or CCM3 (PDCD10), MAP3K3, PIK3CA, and MAP2K7	Somatic mosaicism	Deep vascular gene panel
Sporadic capillary malformations	GNA11, GNAQ, PIK3CA, PIK3R1, and AKT3	Somatic mosaicism	Deep vascular gene panel
Sturge Weber syndrome	GNAQ, GNA11	Somatic mosaicism	Deep vascular gene panel
Gorham Stout disease	KRAS	Somatic mosaicism	Deep vascular gene panel
Generalized lymphatic anomaly	PIK3CA	Somatic mosaicism	Deep vascular gene panel
Kaposiform lymphangiomatosis	NRAS, CBL, HRAS, and PIK3CA	Somatic mosaicism	Deep vascular gene panel

For vascular anomalies caused by somatic mosaicism, a deep vascular gene panel should be considered for testing rather than a germline panel. It is important to note that deep vascular gene panels will be able to detect germline variants so it is better to err on the side of deeper coverage if there is a question.
The * indicates cause in case reports.

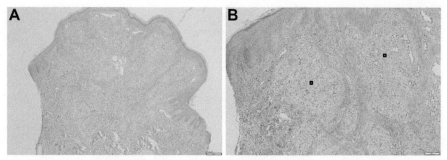

Fig. 4. Pyogenic Granuloma. (*A*) Low power (2 ×) shows a lobular proliferations of capillaries. On the resection edges, the superficial skin epithelium is noted. (*B*) The lobular architecture (4 ×) of the capillary-sized vessels is noted (marked with *square*).

typically caused by pathogenic variants in the RAS-MAPK pathway (see **Fig. 1**).[29]

Arteriovenous Malformations

Loss of the intervening capillary bed between arteries and veins results in an arteriovenous malformation (AVM) leading to direct connection between a fast-flow artery and slow-flow vein. If visible on physical examination, they may be pulsatile masses with or without a blush. AVMs may lead to pain and bleeding. Histologically, there will be features of both thick-walled arteries and thin-walled, ectatic veins (**Fig. 5**). AVMs may be sporadic and caused by mosaic, pathogenic variants in genes that lead to activation of the RAS-MAPK pathway.[31,32] In the brain, the most common cause is *KRAS,* followed by *BRAF.*[33–35] In contrast, AVMs of the body are usually due to *MAP2K1.*[36] Other mosaic causes include *BRAF* and *HRAS.*[37,37] Laser microcapture dissection demonstrated that somatic pathogenic variants are present in the endothelial cells.[38]

AVMs can also be syndromic. AVMs are caused by germline, monoallelic pathogenic variants in *RASA1* or *EPHB4* in capillary malformation—arteriovenous malformation syndrome (CM-AVM1 or CM-AVM2) and typically are associated with a

capillary malformation.[39–42] Germline *RASA1* or rarely mosaic pathogenic variants in *KRAS* cause Parkes Weber syndrome characterized by AVMs with capillary malformation and overgrowth.[43,44] AVMs combined with mucocutaneous telangiectasias and epistaxis are characteristic of hereditary hemorrhagic telangiectasia (HHT), which can have overlap with *EPHB4*-related CM-AVM2.[45] HHT is an autosomal dominant disorder caused by monoallelic pathogenic variants in *ENG, ACVRL1, SMAD4,* and *GDF2.*[46–50] Somatic, second-hit pathogenic variants are found in the vascular malformations in individuals with CM-AVM or HHT.[51,52] Finally, AVMs, usually associated with lipomatous growth, are seen in about 50% of individuals with *PTEN* hamartoma syndrome due to germline, monoallelic pathogenic variants in *PTEN.*[53] Rarely, AVMs may also be seen in the spine in individuals with congenital lipomatous overgrowth with vascular anomalies and epidermal nevi (CLOVES) due to mosaic, pathogenic variants in *PIK3CA.*[54]

SLOW-FLOW VASCULAR MALFORMATIONS

Slow-flow vascular malformations involve vessels with slow flow such as venous, lymphatic, and/or capillary vessels either separately or combined

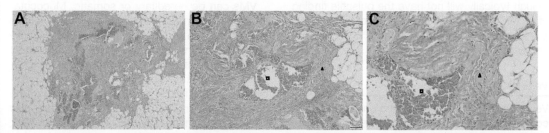

Fig. 5. Arteriovenous malformation. (*A*) Low-power (4 ×) view shows the classical combination of thick-walled and thin-walled vessels. Being subcutaneous, the adipose tissue surrounding the vascular malformation is noted. (*B*) Mid-power (10 ×) and (*C*) High-power (20 ×) views show some ectatic thin-walled veins (marked with *square*) and thick-walled arteries (marked with *triangle*).

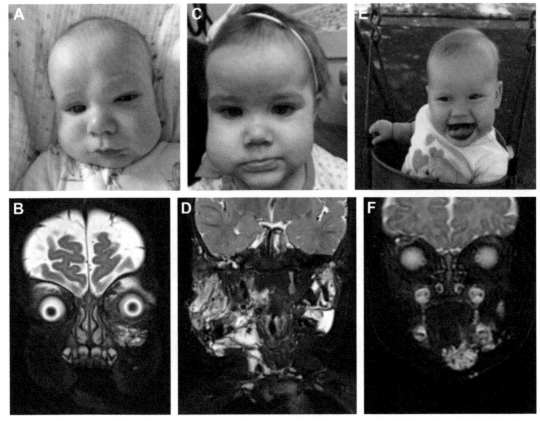

Fig. 6. Photographs and corresponding MRI images of slow-flow head and neck vascular malformations. Patients provided informed written consent for photograph publication. (*A*) Four mo male with left face and orbit macro and microcystic lymphatic malformation. (*B*) MRI T2_tse_fs-dixon of "a" at 5 mo demonstrating large multicystic predominantly T2 hyperintense lesion involving the periorbital and intraorbital as well as the pre malar and buccal soft tissues. (*C*) Twelve mo female with neck and face lymphatic malformation. (*D*) MRI at 15 mo T2_tse_fs-dixon of "c" demonstrates multispatial microcystic and macrocystic lymphatic malformation involving the right more than the left neck and face. (*E*) Lip and face venous malformation. (*F*) MRI of "e" at 3 mo showing T2 hyperintensity and a few small T2 dark pheboliths.

(**Fig. 6**). Slow-flow vascular malformations can be differentiated from fast-flow vascular malformations by the clinical and radiological aspects of the lesion. Slow-flow vascular malformations can present with pain, swelling, psychological distress because of appearance, and functional limitations though typically will not have the pulsatile finding of an AVM. Slow-flow lesions are more commonly caused by components of the PI3K signaling pathway.[56,58,63–65]

Venous Malformation

Venous malformations (VMs) are one of the most common vascular malformations. VMs are congenital malformations but sometimes they are noticed later in life. VM may present as a bluish or purple compressible lesion. When pheloboliths are present, they may present as firm or hard areas in the lesion. VM can lead to pain, swelling, physical deformities, and functional limitations. There can be a solitary or multiple lesions. Histologically, they show dermal lobular proliferation of variably sized and ectatic thin-walled blood vessels (**Fig. 7**).

VMs can be hereditary or somatic. Mucocutaneous venous malformations present with multiple VMs on the skin and mucous membranes with variable sizes, dome-shaped with a bluish coloration. Mucocutaneous venous malformations are a hereditary presentation caused by monoallelic pathogenic variants in *TEK*, which encodes the tyrosine kinase receptor TIE2.[55] Sporadic VMs are also caused by somatic, pathogenic variants in *TEK*; however, some may be due to somatic, pathogenic *PIK3CA* variants.[55–58] Blue rubber bleb nevus syndrome (BRBNS) presents with multiple small characteristic bluish, spongy, compressible

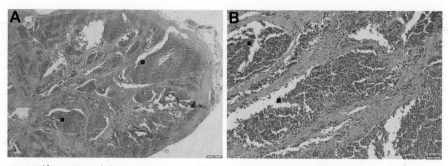

Fig. 7. Venous Malformation. (*A*) Low power (4 ×) shows a dermal lobular proliferation of variably sized and ectatic thin-walled blood vessels (marked with *square*). (*B*) High power (20 ×) demonstrates the thin-walls lining the vessels (marked with *square*), which contain numerous red blood cells.

cutaneous lesions; typically on the hands and feet. BRBNS is caused by somatic, pathogenic variants in the *TEK* gene, and this is typically double-cis (two pathogenic variants present on the same allele).[59]

Lymphatic Malformation

Lymphatic malformations (LMs) are benign vascular malformations of the lymphatic system resulting from dilation or cystic formation in the lymphatic vasculature.[60] Although LMs may present all over the body, most LM cases (75%) reside in the head and neck region due to the greater quantity of lymphatic vessels within this region that do not properly connect and drain into the venous system.[60,61] Cystic LMs are categorized by their size; microcystic if they are too small to undergo sclerotherapy which tends to translate to less than 2 cm in diameter, macrocystic LMs, which tend to be easier to treat and may resolve on their own, or mixed cystic LMs if patients have both microcystic and microcystic LMs.[2,5] Interestingly, microcystic and macrocystic LMs appear similar histologically with dilated lymphatic vessels that may carry amorphous protein-containing fluid situated near lymphoid tissue and adipocytes (**Fig. 8**) and are CD31 positive and D2-40 positive.[5] This finding suggests that the severity of microcystic LMs compared to macrocystic LMs may be caused by factors other than the immunohistochemistry of the tissue, such as anatomic location.[5]

Cystic LMs are typically caused by a somatic, pathogenic activating *PIK3CA* variant that may be detected in the lymphatic endothelial cells (LEC) which line the LM.[62–66] Activation of PIK3CA has been attributed to lymphangiogenic properties including increased LEC sprouting, and vascular endothelial growth factor (VEGF) and cyclooxygenase 2 (COX2) expression, demonstrating how activation of this pathway can lead to a cystic LM phenotype.[62] Additionally, a small number of LMs have been linked to mutations in *PIK3R1, BRAF,* and *KRAS*.[43,67–70]

Mixed Slow-Flow Malformation

The mixed slow-flow malformation is a combined vascular malformation involving at least two vessel types such as capillaries, veins, and/or lymphatics. Mixed slow-flow vascular malformations can be

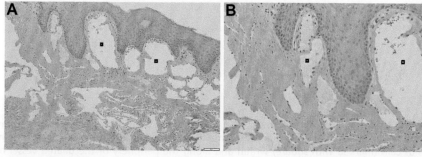

Fig. 8. Lymphatic Malformation. (*A*) Low power (4 ×) shows dilated lymphatic vascular channels with very thin endothelium (marked with *square*) in the papillary dermis in this tongue biopsy. (*B*) In this higher power (20 ×) view, some of the lymphatic channels contain pink, proteinaceous material.

isolated or part of a syndromic presentation such as Klippel–Trenaunay Syndrome with bone and tissue overgrowth.[65] These are typically due to somatic pathogenic variants in *PIK3CA*.[65] Histologically, mixed slow-flow vascular malformations will have combined components of the individual malformations.

Glomuvenous Malformation

Glomuvenous malformations (GVMs) are a hereditary type of cutaneous venous malformation that presents with blue-purple lesions on the skin and mucosal surfaces.[78] It may have a cobblestone raised appearance, feel tender on palpation, and is not easily compressible.[78] GVMs may cause paroxysmal stabbing pain, point tenderness, and cold hypersensitivity because the glomus body oversees regulation of blood flow to the skin and temperature regulation.[78] Histologically, dense venous-like proliferation of dilated blood vessels and glomus cells are seen (**Fig. 9**). GVMs are an autosomal dominant disorder due to monoallelic, pathogenic variants in *GLMN*.[71] The lesions increase in number over time, and arise due to the accumulation of subsequent second hits, usually uniparental isodisomy.[71,72]

Verrucous Venous Malformation

Verrucous venous malformations (VVMs) present as purple and hyperkeratotic linear plaques with a verrucous surface and often get misdiagnosed with other vascular tumors and malformations due to their similar clinical appearance.[73] In younger individuals, VVMs can be non-keratotic, but they become increasingly hyperkeratotic over time.[73] VVM usually involves the epidermis, dermis, and subcutaneous fat.[73] It can present with complications such as bleeding, pain, or functional impairment. VVM is caused by somatic, pathogenic variants in *MAP3K3*.[74]

Cerebral Cavernous Malformation

Cerebral cavernous malformations are vascular malformations that involve the brain and/or spinal cord.[75] The vascular malformation is described as a cavernoma because it comprises closely clustered, enlarged capillary channels mimicking a cavern. Some patients may not have any clinical symptoms, but they have higher risks for stroke, seizures, motor and sensory deficits, and headaches. It usually becomes symptomatic in patients between 20 and 30 years of age. Patients can also present with cutaneous vascular malformations

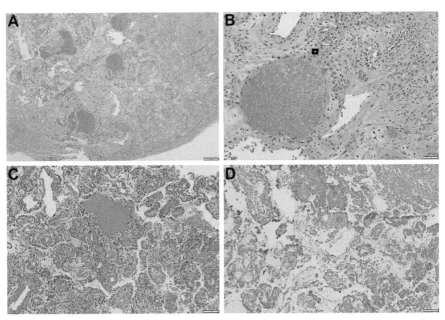

Fig. 9. Glomuvenous Malformation. (*A*) Low-power (4 ×) view of dense venous-like proliferation of dilated blood vessels and glomus cells, composing this glomulovenous malformation. (*B*) High-power (20 ×) view demonstrates clusters of glomus cells (marked with *square*) within and along the periphery of the dilated vessel helping to distinguish it from a venous malformation. (*C*) Middle-power (10 ×) view that demonstrates abundant glomus cells with strong cytoplasmic staining as highlighted in (*D*) by smooth muscle actin (SMA) immunohistochemical stain (brown staining).

concomitantly.[76] Histologically, the malformation is characterized by marked dilation of back-to-back uniform-appearing blood vessels, some of which have thrombus. The reactive brain parenchyma surrounds the malformation (**Fig. 10**). This condition can be hereditary or sporadic. Familial cerebral cavernous malformation is an autosomal dominant condition due to monoallelic pathogenic variants in *CCM1 (KRIT1)*, *CCM2 (MGC4607)*, or *CCM3 (PDCD10)*.[75–77,79–83] Testing for the genetic cause of CCM should always include deletion/duplication analysis as there is a frequently identified exon 2-10 deletion in *CCM2* and a increased percentage of deletion variants in *KRIT1*.[91,92] The sporadic form may also be caused by somatic pathogenic variants in the *CCM1 (KRIT1)*, *CCM2 (MGC4607)*, or *CCM3 (PDCD10)*, *MAP3K3*, *PIK3CA*, and *MAP2K7* genes.[75–77,79–83]

Capillary Malformations

Capillary malformations are the most common VM in neonates, with an estimated occurrence of 0.3%.[40] The term "capillary malformation" acts as a greater categorical term in the classification of birthmarks referring to lesions caused by dilated vessels in the papillary dermis.[4] Histologically, capillary malformations may have increased capillary density, including some ectatic vessels (**Fig. 11**).

Port wine nevi (PWN) are the most common capillary malformation with an occurrence of 0.3% to 0.5% of infants.[93] Because of this, researchers may use the more general term: capillary malformations when referencing PWN. Unlike other conditions categorized as nevi flammeus, capillary malformations typically remain after the first year of life and changes over time may be driven by the genetics, although the size and distribution of the lesion do not change.[94]

Capillary malformations may be isolated or syndromic and caused by somatic, pathogenic variants in *GNA11*, *GNAQ*, *PIK3CA*, *PIK3R1*, and *AKT3*.[67,84–90,95] Capillary malformations may present only with undergrowth or overgrowth. In addition to the growth differences, there may be congenital malformations for example, in individuals with megalencephaly capillary malformation (MCAP) or other *PIK3CA*-related spectrum disorders–or *PIK3R1*-related disorder.[65,67] If the typical philtrum capillary malformation is present in an individual with MCAP, often times a buccal swab between the upper lip and mucosa will be a sufficient affected tissue sample for DNA sample collection. Sturge-Weber Syndrome is characterized by facial capillary malformations, glaucoma,

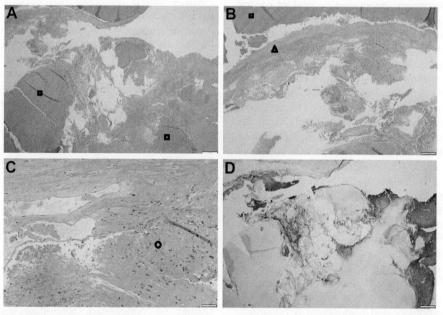

Fig. 10. Brain Cavernoma (Cerebral Cavernous Malformation). (*A*) Low-power (4 ×) view shows marked dilation of back-to-back uniform-appearing blood vessels, some of which have thrombus (marked with *square*). The reactive brain parenchyma surrounds the malformation. (*B*) Mid-power (10 ×) shows partial thrombus and hyalinized blood vessel walls (marked with *triangle*). (*C*) High-power (20 ×) view shows numerous hemosiderin-laden macrophages, foamy histiocytes, and reactive astrocytes (marked with *circle*). (*D*) Immunohistochemical stain for glial fibrillary acidic protein (GFAP) highlights the circumscription of the blood vessel malformation by brain parenchyma (brown staining).

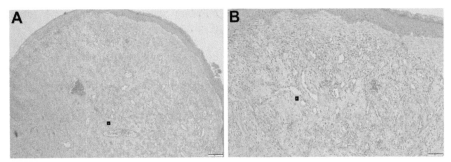

Fig. 11. Capillary Malformation (*A*) Low-power (4 ×) view shows the increased capillary density, some of which are ectatic (marked with *square*), especially in the deeper dermis where they are more prominent. (*B*) Higher power (20 ×) shows ectatic (marked with *square*), thin-walled vessels (lacking smooth muscle) and numerous extravasated red blood cells.

and/or leptomeningeal angiomatosis and is due to mosaic, pathogenic variants in *GNAQ* or *GNA11*.[89,96,97]

Hereditary capillary malformations may also be seen in autosomal dominant disorders such as CM-AVM1 and CM-AVM2 due to monoallelic pathogenic variants in *RASA1* or *EPHB4*.[42,45] While almost all individuals with CM-AVM1 and CM-AVM2 will present with capillary malformations, only a subset will have AVMs.[39,42,45]

COMPLEX LYMPHATIC ANOMALIES

Complex lymphatic anomalies consist of central conducting lymphatic anomaly, Gorham Stout disease, generalized lymphatic anomaly, and Kaposiform lymphangiomatosis. These are a group of four distinct, but overlapping, disorders of lymphatic malformations in bones, organs, and lymphatics. Gorham Stout disease, generalized lymphatic anomaly, and Kaposiform lymphangiomatosis may present with manifestations in the head and neck including lymphatic malformations in the spine. Gorham Stout disease, also known as vanishing bone disease, is characterized by lymphatic proliferation in the bone causing progressive cortical osteolysis. In the head and neck, the skull, especially maxillofacial bones, cervical spine, or temporal bones may be affected.[127,127] This can result in pain, fracture, and cerebrospinal fluid leaks.[127] Gorham stout disease is caused by somatic, pathogenic variants in *KRAS*.[98,99] In contrast to Gorham Stout disease, the lymphatic malformations due to generalized lymphatic anomaly and Kaposiform lymphangiomatosis cause medullary osteolysis. Generalized lymphatic anomaly is caused by somatic, pathogenic variants in *PIK3CA*.[100] Kaposiform lymphangiomatosis is caused by somatic, pathogenic variants in *NRAS, CBL, HRAS,* and *PIK3CA*.[101–104,115,116]

THERAPIES

A full delineation of the medical therapies used to treat vascular anomalies is beyond the scope of this review. However, it is important for all clinicians to understand the impact of genetic testing on medical therapy. The identification of genetic pathway drivers is essential for choosing a pathway inhibitor that targets the activating pathogenic variants driving vascular anomaly pathology.

Landmark studies demonstrated that sirolimus, an mTOR inhibitor, is efficacious and safe for most vascular anomalies.[105–114,117] More recently, the discovery of alpelisib for the treatment of *PIK3CA*-related disorders has transformed the field, though clinical trials are still ongoing.[118–121] Alpelisib treatment may also be efficacious for *PIK3R1*-related disorders as well, though further research is needed. MEK inhibitors, such as trametinib and selumetinib, have been used in individual case studies for treatment of arteriovenous malformations and complex lymphatic anomalies due to activating pathogenic variants in the RAS-MAPK pathway.[31,103,104,122–130] Clinical trials evaluating the efficacy of MEK inhibition are ongoing for treatment of AVMs and under development for complex lymphatic anomalies.

SUMMARY

In conclusion, genetic evaluation is an essential component of refining the diagnosis of the vascular anomaly. When sending genetic testing, the type of DNA, the type of sample, and the coverage depth needed to identify the cause should be considered. Slow-flow lesions are more likely to be caused by genes in the PI3K signaling pathway, while fast-flow lesions are more likely to be caused by genes in the RAS-MAPK signaling pathway. Successful identification of the genetic etiology may drive the choice of therapy.

CLINICS CARE POINTS

- Diagnosis of a vascular anomaly is made by history, physical examination, imaging, histology, and genetics all helping to define the lesion.
- If one is unsure if the cause is germline or somatic, sending a somatic panel may ensure adequate depth of coverage to detect a pathogenic variant; however, careful consideration of need to biopsy an affected tissue sample should be considered.
- Cell-free DNA or "liquid biopsy" has recently become available clinically for genetic diagnosis of vascular malformations.
- The genetic cause of a vascular anomaly can direct the type of medical therapy used to treat the anomaly.

ACKNOWLEDGMENTS

The authors thank the patients and their families for use of their participation. The authors thank Alan Hoofring and Ethan Tyler of the NIH Medical Arts Branch for their assistance with **Fig. 1**.

DISCLOSURE

K.M. Woodis, L.D.G. Torales, and S.E. Sheppard wrote the original draft. K.M. Woodis, A. Wolf, A. Britt, and S.E. Sheppard prepared the figures and tables. All authors reviewed and edited the final draft. K.M. Woodis, L.D.G. Torales, and S.E. Sheppard are supported by the *Eunice Kennedy Shriver* National Institute of Child Health and Human Development, United States under award number ZIA-HD009003-01. The content is solely the responsibility of the authors and does not necessarily represent the official views of the National Institutes of Health. The authors have no conflicts of interest to declare.

REFERENCES

1. Tasnádi G. Hemangiomas and Vascular Malformations, An Atlas of Diagnosis and Treatment. 2009; 109–10.
2. Wassef M, Blei F, Adams D, et al. Vascular anomalies classification: recommendations from the international society for the study of vascular anomalies. Pediatrics 2015;136(1):e203–14.
3. Funaki B, Funaki C. Embolization of high-flow arteriovenous malformation. Semin Intervent Rad 2016; 33(02):157–60.
4. Happle R. Capillary malformations: a classification using specific names for specific skin disorders. J Eur Acad Dermatol 2015;29(12):2295–305.
5. Chen EY, Hostikka SL, Oliaei S, et al. Similar histologic features and immunohistochemical staining in microcystic and macrocystic lymphatic malformations. Lymphat Res Biol 2009;7(2):75–80.
6. Thorpe J, Osei-Owusu IA, Avigdor BE, et al. Mosaicism in human health and disease. Annu Rev Genet 2020;54(1):1–24.
7. Li D, Sheppard SE, March ME, et al. Genomic profiling informs diagnoses and treatment in vascular anomalies. Nat Med 2023. https://doi.org/10.1038/s41591-023-02364-x.
8. Zenner K, Jensen DM, Cook TT, et al. Cell-free DNA as a diagnostic analyte for molecular diagnosis of vascular malformations. Genetics Medicine Official J Am Coll Medical Genetics 2021;23(1):123–30.
9. Serio VB, Palmieri M, Loberti L, et al. Nosological and theranostic approach to vascular malformation through cfdna ngs liquid biopsy. J Clin Medicine 2022;11(13):3740.
10. Palmieri M, Sarno LD, Tommasi A, et al. MET somatic activating mutations are responsible for lymphovenous malformation and can be identified using cell-free DNA next generation sequencing liquid biopsy. J Vasc Surg Venous Lymphatic Disord 2021;9(3):740–4.
11. Palmieri M, Currò A, Tommasi A, et al. Cell-free DNA next-generation sequencing liquid biopsy as a new revolutionary approach for arteriovenous malformation. Jvs-vascular Sci 2020;1:176–80.
12. Palmieri M, Pinto AM, Blasio L di, et al. A pilot study of next generation sequencing–liquid biopsy on cell-free DNA as a novel non-invasive diagnostic tool for Klippel–Trenaunay syndrome. Vascular 2021;29(1):85–91.
13. Seattle Children's Hospital. 2023. SpotSeq ddPCR. https://seattlechildrenslab.testcatalog.org/show/LAB3822-1.
14. McDonough SJ, Bhagwate A, Sun Z, et al. Use of FFPE-derived DNA in next generation sequencing: DNA extraction methods. PLoS One 2019;14(4): e0211400.
15. McNulty SN, Evenson MJ, Corliss MM, et al. Diagnostic utility of next-generation sequencing for disorders of somatic mosaicism: a five-year cumulative cohort. Am J Hum Genetics 2019; 105(4):734–46.
16. Siegel DH, Cottrell CE, Streicher JL, et al. Analyzing the genetic spectrum of vascular anomalies with overgrowth via cancer genomics. J Invest Dermatol 2018;138(4):957–67.
17. Dickison P, Christou E, Wargon O. A prospective study of infantile hemangiomas with a focus on incidence and risk factors. Pediatr Dermatol 2011; 28(6):663–9.

18. Bandera AIR, Sebaratnam DF, Wargon O, et al. Infantile hemangioma. Part 1: Epidemiology, pathogenesis, clinical presentation and assessment. J Am Acad Dermatol 2021;85(6):1379–92.

19. Metry D, Heyer G, Hess C, et al. Consensus statement on diagnostic criteria for PHACE syndrome. Pediatrics 2009;124(5):1447–56.

20. Cotton CH, Ahluwalia J, Balkin DM, et al. Association of demographic factors and infantile hemangioma characteristics with risk of PHACE syndrome. Jama Dermatol 2021;157(8):932–9.

21. Garzon MC, Epstein LG, Heyer GL, et al. PHACE Syndrome: Consensus-Derived Diagnosis and Care Recommendations. J Pediatr 2016;178: 24–33.e2.

22. Haggstrom AN, Garzon MC, Baselga E, et al. Risk for PHACE Syndrome in Infants With Large Facial Hemangiomas. Pediatrics 2010;126(2):e418–26.

23. Siegel DH. PHACE syndrome: Infantile hemangiomas associated with multiple congenital anomalies: Clues to the cause. Am J Med Genet Part C Seminars Medical Genetics 2018;178(4):407–13.

24. Jafarzadeh H, Sanatkhani M, Mohtasham N. Oral pyogenic granuloma: a review. J Oral Sci 2006; 48(4):167–75.

25. Groesser L, Peterhof E, Evert M, et al. BRAF and RAS Mutations in Sporadic and Secondary Pyogenic Granuloma. J Invest Dermatol 2016;136(2): 481–6.

26. dos Santos Fontes Pereira T, Amorim LSD, Pereira NB, et al. Oral pyogenic granulomas show MAPK/ERK signaling pathway activation, which occurs independently of BRAF, KRAS, HRAS, NRAS, GNA11, and GNA14 mutations. J Oral Pathol Med 2019;48(10):906–10.

27. Lim YH, Bacchiocchi A, Qiu J, et al. GNA14 somatic mutation causes congenital and sporadic vascular tumors by MAPK Activation. Am J Hum Genetics 2016;99(2):443–50.

28. Broek RWT, Koelsche C, Eijkelenboom A, et al. Kaposiform hemangioendothelioma and tufted angioma – (epi)genetic analysis including genome-wide methylation profiling. Ann Diagn Pathol 2020;44:151434.

29. Al-Olabi L, Polubothu S, Dowsett K, et al. Mosaic RAS/MAPK variants cause sporadic vascular malformations which respond to targeted therapy. J Clin Invest 2018;128(4):1496–508.

30. Lyons LL, North PE, Lai FM-M, et al. Kaposiform Hemangioendothelioma. Am J Surg Pathol 2004; 28(5):559–68.

31. Smits PJ, Konczyk DJ, Sudduth CL, et al. Endothelial MAP2K1 mutations in arteriovenous malformation activate the RAS/MAPK pathway. Biochem Bioph Res Co 2020;529(2):450–4.

32. Fish JE, Suarez CPF, Boudreau E, et al. Somatic Gain of KRAS Function in the Endothelium Is Sufficient to Cause Vascular Malformations That Require MEK but Not PI3K Signaling. Circ Res 2020;127(6):727–43.

33. Goss JA, Huang AY, Smith E, et al. Somatic mutations in intracranial arteriovenous malformations. PLoS One 2019;14(12):e0226852.

34. Nikolaev SI, Vetiska S, Bonilla X, et al. Somatic Activating KRAS Mutations in Arteriovenous Malformations of the Brain. N Engl J Med 2018;378(3): 250–61.

35. Hong T, Yan Y, Li J, et al. High prevalence of KRAS/BRAF somatic mutations in brain and spinal cord arteriovenous malformations. Brain 2018;142(1): 23–34.

36. Couto JA, Huang AY, Konczyk DJ, et al. Somatic MAP2K1 Mutations Are Associated with Extracranial Arteriovenous Malformation. Am J Hum Genetics 2017;100(3):546–54.

37. Konczyk DJ, Goss JA, Smits PJ, et al. Arteriovenous malformation associated with a HRAS mutation. Hum Genet 2019;138(11–12):1419–21.

38. Konczyk DJ, Goss JA, Smits PJ, et al. Arteriovenous Malformation MAP2K1 Mutation Causes Local Cartilage Overgrowth by a Cell-Non Autonomous Mechanism. Sci Rep-uk 2020;10(1):4428.

39. Amyere M, Revencu N, Helaers R, et al. Germline Loss-of-Function Mutations in EPHB4 Cause a Second Form of Capillary Malformation-Arteriovenous Malformation (CM-AVM2) Deregulating RAS-MAPK Signaling. Circulation 2017;136(11):1037–48.

40. Eerola I, Boon LM, Mulliken JB, et al. Capillary Malformation–Arteriovenous Malformation, a New Clinical and Genetic Disorder Caused by RASA1 Mutations. Am J Hum Genetics 2003;73(6):1240–9.

41. Revencu N, Fastre E, Ravoet M, et al. RASA1 mosaic mutations in patients with capillary malformation-arteriovenous malformation. J Med Genet 2020;57(1):48.

42. Revencu N, Boon LM, Mendola A, et al. RASA1 Mutations and Associated Phenotypes in 68 Families with Capillary Malformation–Arteriovenous Malformation. Hum Mutat 2013;34(12):1632–41.

43. Eng W, Sudduth CL, Konczyk DJ, et al. Parkes Weber Syndrome with Lymphedema Caused by a Somatic KRAS Variant. Mol Case Stud 2021;7(6): a006118.

44. Revencu N, Boon LM, Mulliken JB, et al. Parkes Weber syndrome, vein of Galen aneurysmal malformation, and other fast-flow vascular anomalies are caused by RASA1 mutations. Hum Mutat 2008; 29(7):959–65.

45. Wooderchak-Donahue WL, Akay G, Whitehead K, et al. Phenotype of CM-AVM2 caused by variants in EPHB4: how much overlap with hereditary hemorrhagic telangiectasia (HHT)? Genet Med 2019; 21(9):2007–14.

46. McAllister KA, Grogg KM, Johnson DW, et al. Endoglin, a TGF-β binding protein of endothelial cells,

is the gene for hereditary haemorrhagic telangiectasia type 1. Nat Genet 1994;8(4):345–51.

47. Wooderchak-Donahue WL, McDonald J, O'Fallon B, et al. BMP9 Mutations Cause a Vascular-Anomaly Syndrome with Phenotypic Overlap with Hereditary Hemorrhagic Telangiectasia. Am J Hum Genetics 2013;93(3):530–7.

48. Johnson DW, Berg JN, Baldwin MA, et al. Mutations in the activin receptor–like kinase 1 gene in hereditary haemorrhagic telangiectasia type 2. Nat Genet 1996;13(2):189–95.

49. Urness LD, Sorensen LK, Li DY. Arteriovenous malformations in mice lacking activin receptor-like kinase-1. Nat Genet 2000;26(3):328–31.

50. Gallione CJ, Richards JA, Letteboer TGW, et al. SMAD4 mutations found in unselected HHT patients. J Med Genet 2006;43(10):793.

51. Lapinski PE, Doosti A, Salato V, et al. Somatic second hit mutation of RASA1 in vascular endothelial cells in capillary malformation-arteriovenous malformation. Eur J Med Genet 2018;61(1):11–6.

52. Snellings DA, Gallione CJ, Clark DS, et al. Somatic Mutations in Vascular Malformations of Hereditary Hemorrhagic Telangiectasia Result in Bi-allelic Loss of ENG or ACVRL1. Am J Hum Genetics 2019;105(5):894–906.

53. Tan W-H, Baris HN, Burrows PE, et al. The spectrum of vascular anomalies in patients with PTEN mutations: implications for diagnosis and management. J Med Genet 2007;44(9):594.

54. Alomari AI, Chaudry G, Rodesch G, et al. Complex Spinal-Paraspinal Fast-Flow Lesions in CLOVES Syndrome: Analysis of Clinical and Imaging Findings in 6 Patients. Am J Neuroradiol 2011;32(10):1812–7.

55. Limaye N, Wouters V, Uebelhoer M, et al. Somatic mutations in angiopoietin receptor gene TEK cause solitary and multiple sporadic venous malformations. Nat Genet 2009;41(1):118–24.

56. Castel P, Carmona FJ, Grego-Bessa J, et al. Somatic PIK3CA mutations as a driver of sporadic venous malformations. Sci Transl Med 2016;8(332):332ra42.

57. Soblet J, Limaye N, Uebelhoer M, et al. Variable Somatic TIE2 Mutations in Half of Sporadic Venous Malformations. Mol Syndromol 2013;4(4):179–83.

58. Limaye N, Kangas J, Mendola A, et al. Somatic Activating PIK3CA Mutations Cause Venous Malformation. Am J Hum Genetics 2015;97(6):914–21.

59. Soblet J, Kangas J, Nätynki M, et al. Blue Rubber Bleb Nevus (BRBN) Syndrome Is Caused by Somatic TEK (TIE2) Mutations. J Invest Dermatol 2017;137(1):207–16.

60. Dubois J, Thomas-Chaussé F, Soulez G. Common (Cystic) Lymphatic Malformations: Current Knowledge and Management. Tech Vasc Intervent Radiol 2019;22(4):100631.

61. Elluru RG, Balakrishnan K, Padua HM. Lymphatic malformations: Diagnosis and management. Semin Pediatr Surg 2014;23(4):178–85.

62. Osborn AJ, Dickie P, Neilson DE, et al. Activating PIK3CA alleles and lymphangiogenic phenotype of lymphatic endothelial cells isolated from lymphatic malformations. Hum Mol Genet 2015;24(4):926–38.

63. Zenner K, Cheng CV, Jensen DM, et al. Genotype correlates with clinical severity in PIK3CA-associated lymphatic malformations. JCI Insight 2019;4(21).

64. Shaheen MF, Tse JY, Sokol ES, et al. Genomic landscape of lymphatic malformations: a case series and response to the PI3Kα inhibitor alpelisib in an N-of-1 clinical trial. Elife 2022;11:e74510.

65. Luks VL, Kamitaki N, Vivero MP, et al. Lymphatic and Other Vascular Malformative/Overgrowth Disorders Are Caused by Somatic Mutations in PIK3CA. J Pediatr 2015;166(4):1048–54.e5.

66. Blesinger H, Kaulfuß S, Aung T, et al. PIK3CA mutations are specifically localized to lymphatic endothelial cells of lymphatic malformations. PLoS One 2018;13(7):e0200343.

67. Cottrell CE, Bender NR, Zimmermann MT, et al. Somatic PIK3R1 variation as a cause of vascular malformations and overgrowth. Genet Med 2021;23(10):1882–8.

68. Zenner K, Jensen DM, Dmyterko V, et al. Somatic activating BRAF variants cause isolated lymphatic malformations. Hum Genetics Genom Adv 2022;3(2):100101.

69. Lihua J, Feng G, Shanshan M, et al. Somatic KRAS mutation in an infant with linear nevus sebaceous syndrome associated with lymphatic malformations. Medicine 2017;96(47):e8016.

70. Sheppard SE, March ME, Seiler C, et al. Lymphatic disorders caused by mosaic, activating KRAS variants respond to MEK inhibition. Jci Insight 2023;8(9).

71. Brouillard P, Boon LM, Mulliken JB, et al. Mutations in a Novel Factor, Glomulin, Are Responsible for Glomuvenous Malformations ("Glomangiomas"). Am J Hum Genetics 2002;70(4):866–74.

72. Amyere M, Aerts V, Brouillard P, et al. Somatic Uniparental Isodisomy Explains Multifocality of Glomuvenous Malformations. Am J Hum Genetics 2013;92(2):188–96.

73. Boccara O, Ariche-Maman S, Hadj-Rabia S, et al. Verrucous hemangioma (also known as verrucous venous malformation): A vascular anomaly frequently misdiagnosed as a lymphatic malformation. Pediatr Dermatol 2018;35(6):e378–81.

74. Couto JA, Vivero MP, Kozakewich HPW, et al. A Somatic MAP3K3 Mutation Is Associated with Verrucous Venous Malformation. Am J Hum Genetics 2015;96(3):480–6.

75. Gault J, Sain S, Hu L-J, et al. Spectrum Of Genotype And Clinical Manifestations In Cerebral Cavernous Malformations. Neurosurgery 2006;59(6):1278–85.

76. Sirvente J, Enjolras O, Wassef M, et al. Frequency and phenotypes of cutaneous vascular malformations in a consecutive series of 417 patients with familial cerebral cavernous malformations. J Eur Acad Dermatol 2009;23(9):1066–72.

77. Zhou Z, Tang AT, Wong W-Y, et al. Cerebral cavernous malformations arise from endothelial gain of MEKK3–KLF2/4 signalling. Nature 2016; 532(7597):122–6.

78. Boon LM, Mulliken JB, Enjolras O, Vikkula M. Glomuvenous malformation (glomangioma) and venous malformation: distinct clinicopathologic and genetic entities. Arch Dermatol 2004;140(8):971–6.

79. Akers AL, Johnson E, Steinberg GK, et al. Biallelic somatic and germline mutations in cerebral cavernous malformations (CCMs): evidence for a two-hit mechanism of CCM pathogenesis. Hum Mol Genet 2009;18(5):919–30.

80. Gault J, Shenkar R, Recksiek P, et al. Biallelic Somatic and Germ Line CCM1 Truncating Mutations in a Cerebral Cavernous Malformation Lesion. Stroke 2005;36(4):872–4.

81. Sahoo T, Johnson EW, Thomas JW, et al. Mutations in the Gene Encoding KRIT1, a Krev-1/rap1a Binding Protein, Cause Cerebral Cavernous Malformations (CCM1). Hum Mol Genet 1999;8(12):2325–33.

82. Liquori CL, Berg MJ, Siegel AM, et al. Mutations in a Gene Encoding a Novel Protein Containing a Phosphotyrosine-Binding Domain Cause Type 2 Cerebral Cavernous Malformations. Am J Hum Genetics 2003;73(6):1459–64.

83. Couteulx SL, Jung HH, Labauge P, et al. Truncating mutations in CCM1, encoding KRIT1, cause hereditary cavernous angiomas. Nat Genet 1999;23(2): 189–93.

84. Couto JA, Ayturk UM, Konczyk DJ, et al. A somatic GNA11 mutation is associated with extremity capillary malformation and overgrowth. Angiogenesis 2017;20(3):303–6.

85. Bolli A, Nriagu B, Britt AD, et al. Mosaic pathogenic variants in AKT3 cause capillary malformation and undergrowth. Am J Med Genet 2023;191(5): 1442–6.

86. Jordan M, Carmignac V, Sorlin A, et al. Reverse phenotyping in patients with skin capillary malformations and mosaic GNAQ or GNA11 mutations defines a clinical spectrum with genotype-phenotype correlation. J Invest Dermatol 2019; 140(5):1106–10.e2.

87. Ayturk UM, Couto JA, Hann S, et al. Somatic Activating Mutations in GNAQ and GNA11 Are Associated with Congenital Hemangioma. Am J Hum Genetics 2016;98(6):1271.

88. Galeffi F, Snellings DA, Wetzel-Strong SE, et al. A novel somatic mutation in GNAQ in a capillary malformation provides insight into molecular pathogenesis. Angiogenesis 2022;25(4):493–502.

89. Shirley MD, Tang H, Gallione CJ, et al. Sturge–Weber Syndrome and Port-Wine Stains Caused by Somatic Mutation in GNAQ. N Engl J Med 2013;368(21):1971–9.

90. Cubiró X, Rozas-Muñoz E, Castel P, et al. Clinical and genetic evaluation of six children with diffuse capillary malformation and undergrowth. Pediatr Dermatol 2020;37(5):833–8.

91. Liquori CL, Berg MJ, Squitieri F, et al. Deletions in CCM2 are a common cause of cerebral cavernous malformations. Am J Hum Genet 2007;80(1):69–75.

92. Riant F, Bergametti F, Fournier HD, et al. CCM3 Mutations Are Associated with Early-Onset Cerebral Hemorrhage and Multiple Meningiomas. Mol Syndromol 2013;4(4):165–72.

93. Chen JK, Ghasri P, Aguilar G, et al. An overview of clinical and experimental treatment modalities for port wine stains. J Am Acad Dermatol 2012;67(2): 289–304.

94. Barsky SH, Rosen S, Geer DE, Noe JM. The nature and evolution of port wine stains: a computer-assisted study. J Invest Dermatol 1980;74(3):154–7.

95. Martinez-Glez V, Rodriguez-Laguna L, Viana-Huete V, et al. Segmental undergrowth is associated with pathogenic variants in vascular malformation genes: A retrospective case-series study. Clin Genet 2022;101(3):296–306.

96. Polubothu S, A-Olabi L, Boente MC del, et al. GNA11 mutation as a cause of Sturge Weber Syndrome - expansion of the phenotypic spectrum of G-protein related mosaicism and the associated clinical diagnoses. J Invest Dermatol 2019;140(5):1110–3.

97. Dompmartin A, Vleuten CJM, Dekeuleneer V, et al. GNA11-mutated Sturge–Weber syndrome has distinct neurological and dermatological features. Eur J Neurol 2022;29(10):3061–70.

98. Nozawa A, Ozeki M, Niihori T, et al. A somatic activating KRAS variant identified in an affected lesion of a patient with Gorham–Stout disease. J Hum Genet 2020;65(11):995–1001.

99. Sepehr NH, McCarter AL, Helaers R, et al. KRAS-driven model of Gorham-Stout disease effectively treated with trametinib. Jci Insight 2021;6(15): e149831.

100. Rodriguez-Laguna L, Agra N, Ibañez K, et al. Somatic activating mutations in PIK3CA cause generalized lymphatic anomaly. J Exp Med 2019;216(2): 407–18.

101. Barclay SF, Inman KW, Luks VL, et al. A Somatic Activating NRAS Variant Associated with Kaposiform Lymphangiomatosis. Genetics Medicine Official J Am Coll Medical Genetics 2019;21(7):1517–24.

102. Allen-Rhoades W, Al-Ibraheemi A, Kohorst M, et al. Cellular variant of kaposiform lymphangiomatosis: a report of three cases, expanding the morphologic and molecular genetic spectrum of this rare entity. Hum Pathol 2022;122:72–81.

103. Foster JB, Li D, March ME, et al. Kaposiform lymphangiomatosis effectively treated with MEK inhibition. EMBO Mol Med 2020;12(10):e12324.

104. Chowers G, Abebe-Campino G, Golan H, et al. Treatment of severe Kaposiform lymphangiomatosis positive for NRAS mutation by MEK inhibition. Pediatr Res 2022;1–5.

105. Engel ER, Hammill A, Adams D, et al. Response to sirolimus in capillary lymphatic venous malformations and associated syndromes: Impact on symptomatology, quality of life, and radiographic response. Pediatr Blood Cancer 2023;70(4):e30215.

106. Hammill AM, Wentzel M, Gupta A, et al. Sirolimus for the treatment of complicated vascular anomalies in children. Pediatr Blood Cancer 2011;57(6): 1018–24.

107. Adams DM, Trenor CC, Hammill AM, et al. Efficacy and Safety of Sirolimus in the Treatment of Complicated Vascular Anomalies. Pediatrics 2016;137(2): e20153257.

108. Ricci KW, Hammill AM, Mobberley-Schuman P, et al. Efficacy of systemic sirolimus in the treatment of generalized lymphatic anomaly and Gorham–Stout disease. Pediatr Blood Cancer 2019;66(5): e27614.

109. Triana P, Dore M, Cerezo V, et al. Sirolimus in the Treatment of Vascular Anomalies. Eur J Pediatr Surg 2016;27(01):086–90.

110. Maruani A, Tavernier E, Boccara O, et al. Sirolimus (Rapamycin) for Slow-Flow Malformations in Children. Jama Dermatol 2021;157(11):1289–98.

111. Zhou J, Yang K, Chen S, et al. Sirolimus in the treatment of kaposiform lymphangiomatosis. Orphanet J Rare Dis 2021;16(1):260.

112. Hammer J, Seront E, Duez S, et al. Sirolimus is efficacious in treatment for extensive and/or complex slow-flow vascular malformations: a monocentric prospective phase II study. Orphanet J Rare Dis 2018;13(1):191.

113. Sebold AJ, Day AM, Ewen J, et al. Sirolimus Treatment in Sturge-Weber Syndrome. Pediatr Neurol 2021;115:29–40.

114. Ozeki M, Nozawa A, Yasue S, et al. The impact of sirolimus therapy on lesion size, clinical symptoms, and quality of life of patients with lymphatic anomalies. Orphanet J Rare Dis 2019;14(1):141.

115. Li D, March ME, Gutierrez-Uzquiza A, et al. ARAF recurrent mutation causes central conducting lymphatic anomaly treatable with a MEK inhibitor. Nat Med 2019;25(7):1116–22.

116. Grenier JM, Borst AJ, Sheppard SE, et al. Pathogenic variants in PIK3CA are associated with clinical phenotypes of kaposiform lymphangiomatosis, generalized lymphatic anomaly, and central conducting lymphatic anomaly. Pediatr Blood Cancer 2023. e30419.

117. Wiegand S, Wichmann G, Dietz A. Treatment of Lymphatic Malformations with the mTOR Inhibitor Sirolimus: A Systematic Review. Lymphat Res Biol 2018;16(4):330–9.

118. Delestre F, Venot Q, Bayard C, et al. Alpelisib administration reduced lymphatic malformations in a mouse model and in patients. Sci Transl Med 2021;13(614):eabg0809.

119. Venot Q, Blanc T, Rabia SH, et al. Targeted therapy in patients with PIK3CA-related overgrowth syndrome. Nature 2018;558(7711):540–6.

120. Wenger TL, Ganti S, Bull C, et al. Alpelisib for the treatment of PIK3CA-related head and neck lymphatic malformations and overgrowth. Genet Med 2022;24(11):2318–28.

121. Raghavendran P, Albers SE, Phillips JD, et al. Clinical Response to PI3K-α Inhibition in a Cohort of Children and Adults With PIK3CA-Related Overgrowth Spectrum Disorders. J Vasc Anomalies 2022;3(1):e038.

122. Cooke DL, Frieden IJ, Shimano KA. Angiographic Evidence of Response to Trametinib Therapy for a Spinal Cord Arteriovenous Malformation. J Vasc Anomalies 2021;2(3):e018.

123. Gordon K, Moore M, Zanten MV, et al. Case Report: Progressive central conducting lymphatic abnormalities in the RASopathies. Two case reports, including successful treatment by MEK inhibition. Front Genet 2022;13:1001105.

124. Dori Y, Smith C, Pinto E, et al. Severe Lymphatic Disorder Resolved With MEK Inhibition in a Patient With Noonan Syndrome and SOS1 Mutation. Pediatrics 2020;146(6). e20200167.

125. Nakano TA, Rankin AW, Annam A, et al. Trametinib for Refractory Chylous Effusions and Systemic Complications in Children with Noonan Syndrome. J Pediatr 2022;248. 81–88.e1.

126. Nicholson CL, Flanagan S, Murati M, et al. Successful management of an arteriovenous malformation with trametinib in a patient with capillary-malformation arteriovenous malformation syndrome and cardiac compromise. Pediatr Dermatol 2022;39(2):316–9.

127. Edwards EA, Phelps AS, Cooke D, et al. Monitoring Arteriovenous Malformation Response to Genotype-Targeted Therapy. Pediatrics 2020;146(3). e20193206.

128. Sansare K, Saalim M, Jogdand M, et al. Radiographic extent of maxillofacial Gorham's disease and its impact on recurrence: A systematic review. Oral Surg Oral Med Oral Pathol Oral Radiol 2021; 132(1):80–92.

129. Rana I, Buonuomo PS, Mastrogiorgio G, et al. Expanding the spectrum of Gorham Stout disease exploring a single center pediatric case series. Lymphology 2021;54(4):182–94.

130. Yokoi H, Chakravarthy V, Whiting B, et al. Gorham-Stout disease of the spine presenting with intracranial hypotension and cerebrospinal fluid leak: A case report and review of the literature. Surg Neurol Int 2020;11:466.

Lasers and Nonsurgical Modalities

Rishabh Rattan, DDS[a], Nadia Mezghani, DDS[b], Arshad Kaleem, DDS, MD[c], James C. Melville, DDS[d],*

KEYWORDS

- Lasers • Vascular malformation • Hemangiomas • AV malformations • Technology

KEY POINTS

- The maxillofacial surgeon commonly encounters vascular pathology in the head and neck region such as hemangiomas, telangiectasia, and venous malformations.
- Surgical management of vascular anomalies in the head and neck region poses unique challenges in terms of accessibility and selectivity of the diseased tissue.
- Laser therapy has gained attention as an adjunct to surgical measures in the management of vascular pathology in this region for its ability to access and target selective tissue while maintaining the surrounding healthy tissue.
- Laser therapy may allow for a superior patient perioperative experience and minimal postoperative pain and recovery time when compared with the surgical management of such lesions.

INTRODUCTION

The maxillofacial surgeon will routinely encounter and manage pathology of the vasculature found in the head and neck region and will by default treat such pathology by surgical means. Nonsurgical treatment modalities, however, have emerged as both promising alternatives and adjunctive measures in the management of head and neck vasculature anomalies (**Fig. 1**). Some of the most notable and emerging nonsurgical methods in practice today include drug therapies, medical lasers, image-guided embolization, and sclerotherapy. A combination of the aforementioned techniques, with or without a surgical component, is beginning to gain popularity in achieving an optimized clinical response when compared with surgery alone.

Given that the head and neck region is home to some of the most complex and delicate vasculature confined in such a small space when compared

with any other region of the human body, the use of laser therapy in this region may be one of the most exciting emerging nonsurgical tools. Laser therapy allows the skillful surgeon to selectively target the diseased tissue while leaving the healthy tissue untouched, allowing for a much more conservative approach than standard surgical measures. Of course, every emerging medical tool comes with its laybacks; medical lasers as we know of today do not adequately penetrate the deeper tissues, making them a less useful tool when targeting the deep vessels of the head and neck. However, when used for appropriately indicated cases, laser therapy can provide superior cosmetic results without foregoing treatment outcomes. In addition, this treatment modality has proven to be a generally safe and comfortable procedure for not only the patient but the surgeon as well.

This article focuses on laser therapy, not as an all-in-one replacement for surgical procedures,

[a] Bernard & Gloria Pepper Katz Department of Oral & Maxillofacial Surgery, University of Texas Health Science Center at Houston; [b] Oral and Maxillofacial Surgery, Mount Sinai Health System and Jacobi Medical Center; [c] El Paso Head & Neck and Microvascular Surgery, El Paso, TX, USA; [d] Bernard & Gloria Pepper Katz Department of Oral & Maxillofacial Surgery, Oral, Head & Neck Oncology and Microvascular Reconstructive Surgery, University of Texas Health Science Center at Houston, 7500 Cambridge Street Suite 6510, Houston, TX 77054, USA
* Corresponding author. 4902 Fern Street, Bellaire, TX 77401.
E-mail address: James.C.Melville@uth.tmc.edu

Oral Maxillofacial Surg Clin N Am 36 (2024) 19–28
https://doi.org/10.1016/j.coms.2023.09.005

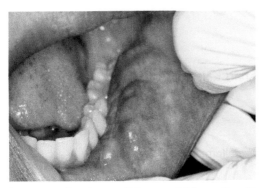

Fig. 1. Vascular abnormalities are visible on the skin surface. (*From* Tran, H.Q., Manon, V.A., Young, S., Melville, J.C. (2022). Lasers and Nonsurgical Modalities. In: Nair, S.C., Chandra, S.R. (eds) Management of Head and Neck Vascular Lesions. Springer, Singapore. https://doi.org/10.1007/978-981-15-2321-2_10.)

but instead as an emerging tool that is quickly being adapted in the management of vascular lesions, particularly in maxillofacial surgery. The authors aim to describe the current state of medical lasers in this field, paying particular attention to their biophysics, clinical uses, and shortcomings. Nonsurgical adjuncts to laser therapy will also be discussed to comprehensively describe its realistic clinical application.

HISTORY OF LASER AND CURRENT MODALITIES

Although the fundamental concept of laser generation was popularized by Albert Einstein in 1916 with his "The Quantum Theory of Radiation," the practical application of this theory was not introduced until 1960. Theodore Maiman, an American physicist, discovered the groundbreaking ruby crystal laser, which incorporated a high-intensity lamp to flash-excite native chromium electrons. On return of these chromium electrons to their original energy states, strong red light pulses would be generated resulting in what is now described as the "laser light." With the advent of this laser beam system, laser application in medicine subsequently began to develop over the following decade. Advanced laser systems such as CO_2, argon, and Nd:YAG grew tremendously at first in dermatology but rapidly escalated to other specialties.

Laser surgery was first set forth as a superior method to conventional surgical modalities for vascular lesions due to its thermal conduction. The continuous energy beam emitted by laser diodes would allow for thermal destruction of target tissues while maintaining hemostasis. Despite its advantages in highly vascularized sites, laser

beam surgery was not free of limitations. The continuous high-energy beam was found to cause nonspecific tissue destruction, resulting in damage to healthy tissue and hypertrophic scar formation. It was not until 1981 that this problem was addressed through the discovery of "selective thermolysis" by Anderson and Parrish. This targeted tissue excision revolved around the concept of chromophores: specific wavelengths of light along the absorption spectrum would be managed preoperatively to spare healthy, nonvascular tissue.[1]

In hopes of optimizing the selectivity of thermolysis, the laser was adjusted to be pulsatile in nature with adjustable wavelengths to maximize the targeted tissue's absorption and minimize the competing components' absorption. The time required for the tissue to lose 50% of its heat through diffusion, termed thermal relaxation, was another important component considered in the optimization of early lasers. It was also put forward that the pulse duration (duration of the beam) should be shorter than the thermal relaxation of the tissue in context. This rule ensures the confinement of the energy released by the laser within the targeted tissue and avoids its emission to the surroundings. In addition, the pulse duration must be of adequate duration for the needed thermal energy inside the vessel to obtain effects of clinical value. Although these principles align well with superficial lesions and the smaller vessel types of the head and neck region, they do not exactly apply to larger diameter vessels or those found at greater depths. In such cases, the appropriate depth of penetration may be achieved by adjusting the wavelength and pulse duration for sufficient thermal energy to build up within the vessel lumen.

The first-generation pulsed dye laser (PDL) was developed in the 1980s and produced light at 577 nm. It was introduced as a replacement for argon lasers, both for its increased safety and efficacy in the treatment of superficial vessel anomalies. The modern day PDLs produce light at 585- or 595-nm wavelengths and usually have built-in cooling systems, improving their efficiency and safety in penetrating greater depths while leaving adjacent tissue untouched. The flash lamp portion of the PDL produces yellow light at a particular wavelength by pumping energy through a rhodamine dye dissolved in a solvent. The energy generated is emitted by fiber-optic technology and shows preferential absorption by hemoglobin and oxyhemoglobin, resulting in thermal-induced damage and coagulative activity within the targeted vessel. The approximated thermal relaxation time of such small cutaneous vessels with diameters of less than 100μm is 1 to 5 ms.[2] Depth continues to be a major limitation of modern day PDLs. Melanin in particular is believed to play a role in the laser's inability to penetrate deeper depths because melanin itself absorbs light produced at the same wavelength as the PDL. This should especially be taken into account when using PDLs on patients with darker skin tones (Fitzpatrick skin types IV/V) because these individuals have a greater concentration of melanin. Given such limitations, PDL use is mainly reserved for vascular lesions of no more than 1.2 mm in depth.[3]

In the head and neck region, the PDL is most commonly used in the setting of superficial vascular abnormalities such as capillary malformations (CMs), superficial infantile hemangiomas, and telangiectasias. Although considered a generally low-risk procedure, some common adverse effects of the use of PDLs for small cutaneous anomalies include erythema, edema, and purpura for up to 2 weeks post-operation. The purpura occurs due to red blood cell leakage out of the vessel walls due to the rapid thermal buildup induced by the laser and associated vessel damage. This adverse effect may be minimized or avoided altogether by using a lower peak energy, which is achieved by increasing the PDL. These adjustments result in a slower and less harmful thermal effect that does not precipitate absolute red blood cell leakage; documented events of purpura after the use of long-pulsed lasers are not known in the current literature.[4] Nevertheless, it is imperative that the surgeon reviews these specific adverse effects before moving forward with PDL therapy, given that they are a common reason for patient refusal of treatment.

Frequency-Doubled Q-Switched Nd:YAG/Potassium Titanyl Phosphate Laser (532 nm)

As its name describes, the frequency-doubled, Q-switched Nd:YAG laser or KTP laser produces green light at 532 nm by using frequency-doubling techniques (second harmonic generation). The 532-nm wavelength is easily absorbed by oxyhemoglobin, making it advantageous in its use for laser thermolysis. Laser energy with a 1064-nm wavelength is produced by pumping the Nd:YAG crystal with a diode laser before focusing it onto a potassium titanyl phosphate (KTP) crystal. This technique results in a second light energy whose frequency is doubled and wavelength is halved to 532 nm ($\lambda = v/f$; λ = wavelength, f = frequency, v = velocity of light).

The 532-nm laser functions at a standard pulse duration of 1- to 50-ms fluence, generating energy as great as 40 J/cm^2. Its utility over other lasers in targeting larger vessels is in part due to its longer

pulse duration necessitated by the estimated thermal relaxation of larger vessels (1–10 ms).[5] This phenomenon allows the laser to focus a substantial and effective amount of thermal energy within these larger vessels, specifically those with a diameter greater than 200 nm. The 532-nm laser was also quickly accepted for its malleability regarding pulse duration and fluence, allowing the clinician to carefully adjust such settings to serve the particular clinical case in question.

One of the major drawbacks of the frequency-doubled Nd:YAG is in regard to its activity with competing melanin. The melanin found in skin has better absorption of light at 532 nm compared with 585 nm, resulting in less penetration of the frequency-doubled Nd:YAG laser in skin types with highly concentrated melanin (ie, Fitzpatrick skin types IV and V). When used in such skin types, the laser may result in discoloration and blistering. This laser's competing activity with melanin, along with the need for a lengthy pulse duration, seem to be the basis of such adverse clinical effects. The implementation of a cooling device perioperatively, however, adds a barrier of protection against unexpected skin damage. It should be noted that these cooling devices do not completely remove the risk of such adverse effects, and these lasers persistently carry a higher risk (18%) of scarring than the standard PDLs (3%).[6] Overall, the frequency-doubled Nd:YAG serves as a reliable alternative in patients who fail to appropriately respond to PDL attempts or those hoping to achieve laser therapy with a lessened risk of developing purpura but should be used with caution in those with darker skin tones.

Long-Pulsed Nd:YAG Laser (1064 nm)

The year of 1964 introduced the 1064-nm Nd:YAG laser, which initially its use was reserved for procedures more cosmetic in nature such as hair removal and scar ablation. It was not until 30 years later in which its application for the management of certain vascular abnormalities was set forth. As the name implies, the 1064-nm Nd:YAG laser uses a wavelength of 1064 nm, functioning through a medium of impure yttrium-aluminum-garnet crystal doped by 1% neodymium ions. The 1064-nm Nd:YAG emerged as a drastically advanced laser; its lower level of absorption effectively reduced the laser's activity with competing melanin, allowing it to reach vessels at depths (5–6 mm) that would otherwise be unreachable by previous lasers. Its lessened competition with melanin compared with previous lasers gained its popularity in the management of vessel anomalies in patients with Fitzpatrick skin types IV and V.

The better suited wavelength of this laser in the context of competing melanin, however, comes with unavoidable interactions with hemoglobin and oxyhemoglobin. These molecules absorb light at 1064 nm, adding a level of distraction between the laser and targeted vessels. The clinician may bypass these interactions by increasing the laser fluence as high as 300 J/cm^2 to ensure adequate generation of thermal energy to promote the coagulation within the targeted vessel. The pulse duration can also be appropriately adjusted between 0.1 and 300 ms to minimize damage imposed by the increased thermal energy on the surrounding tissue, doing so also minimizes the risk of purpura development postoperatively.

During routine practice, the laser is brought into direct contact with the cutaneous tissue. The clinician will make either a single or double pass over the target lesion until blanching or shrinkage of the lesion is observed clinically. Additional passes or persistent contact with the cutaneous tissue exposes the skin to probable postoperative damage and should be avoided. The number of passes over the targeted tissue should be kept at a minimum, and the laser itself should be in continuous movement. In practice, the type of lesion should also be considered; a nodular lesion may warrant the use of a glass slide to flatten the lesion and improve the penetrating depth. The location of the lesion is another characteristic to consider; for lesions with difficult accessibility (ie, palate, floor of the mouth), a test tube with a side window, termed the interstitial technique, may ameliorate the clinician's ability to reach the lesion. A 14-gauge angio-catheter is used to inset a fiber-optic cable into the targeted lesion, allowing for more selective delivery of the laser energy.[7,8] This technique in particular helps protect the overlying tissue when ablating thicker lesions or accessing greater depths. It also may reduce the patient's experienced duration of postoperative pain.

The longer pulsed laser provides reliable outcomes in terms of its use in the treatment of hemangiomas and vascular anomalies; it has been shown to result in a 50% improvement in 71.5% to 80% of all treated vascular lesions.[9,10] An additional study reported an absolute clearance rate of 77% in intraoral lesions after one session; persistent lesions were cleared with one or two additional sessions.[11] Although such numbers offer promising results, the safety window of these longer pulsed lasers is rather narrow and must be approached with caution. As with previous lasers, a cooling device can help avoid the laser's possibility of collateral damage such as blistering and scarring. The clinician should conservatively approach its use; short, multiple sessions offer a reduced risk of damaging effects compared with a single aggressive session.

CO₂ Laser (10,600 nm)

Although the human body is composed of 85% H_2O, mucosal tissue consists of an even higher proportion of H_2O, amounting to roughly 95%. This is largely attributed to the tissue's increased vascularity and secretory contents. The CO_2 laser has therefore been considered a reliable method for ablative procedures because of its ability to penetrate water-rich structures. The thermal energy conducted by this type of laser is effective in both excision and hemostasis. Smaller blood vessels with diameters extending to 0.5 mm can be predictably cauterized by this method.[12,13] The CO_2 laser works under two operative modes: focused and defocused. The focused mode is effective in targeted excision, whereas the defocused setting allows for vaporization of tissue in a layer-by-layer fashion. The defocused mode is preferred in the setting of biopsy-proven dysplasia due to its usability and predictable postoperative healing. Despite its practicality, the clinician must take care in accounting for important anatomic structures due to this method's risk of irregular depth penetration, a complication of tissue water content variability. Furthermore, this approach tends to obliterate tissue samples, thereby disabling concurrent biopsy procedures. The focused method in particular may allow for the gathering of intraoperative biopsy specimens; however, adjacent margins may still be altered, although to a lesser degree as compared with the defocused setting. In the use of focused CO_2 laser biopsy, larger margins may be necessary to include healthy tissue margins within the sample submitted for pathology. Nevertheless, one study focusing on the morphologic, histochemical, and immunocytochemical effects showed blisters, erosions, clefts of epithelium, and nuclei changes in samples retrieved via CO_2 laser.[14]

CO_2 laser ablation has advantages in hemostasis, postoperative healing period, and usability, which directly correlates to reduced intraoperative time. This surgical approach creates an immediate hemostatic site that facilitates fibrin clot deposition and maturation. Furthermore, the unique tissue site created by CO_2 laser ablation delays and reduces inflammatory cell infiltrate, thereby resulting in diminished postoperative swelling. With this reduction in inflammation, postoperative pain has also been reported to be reduced in patients undergoing CO_2 laser surgery. This approach also decreases the amount of residual viable myofibroblasts, a cell-type integral in scar contracture. Owing to this unique feature, CO_2 laser has become a mainstay in surgical resection of pathology in the floor of the mouth as well as buccal mucosa. Wounds are left to heal by secondary intention and do not require primary closure or additional dressing application. For these reasons, CO_2 laser ablation has been adopted as a powerful tool in surgical approaches to maxillofacial pathology.

Diode Laser (532, 800, 810, 940, and 980 nm)

One of the most commonly used lasers by maxillofacial surgeons today is the diode laser, not only for its portability and economic unit system but more importantly for its adjustability and practicality. Engineered through a solid-state semiconductor, the light transmitted by this laser can be programmed to have variable intensity and wavelengths. In line with the principle of selective thermolysis, the 532-nm pulsed mode functions in alignment with the PDL and is effective in the management of superficial vascular defects while preserving surrounding tissues. Its differences lie in the diode laser's capability of emitting longer pulsed energy (1–100 ms) in the absence of causing purpura because of its slower rate of vaporization, preventing vessel rupture.[15] The diode laser can also reach deeper vessels when functioning at 800 to 900 nm and 3 to 5 W, all while sustaining a high rate of selectivity for hemoglobin chromophores. These particular parameters are selected for when aiming to penetrate deeper lesions that are resistant to standard PDL or KTP treatment.

The diode laser's adjustable wavelength, power, and pulse duration are the foundation of its practicality in the clinical setting. The laser bypasses the somewhat narrow use of preceding laser therapies and into the realm of more complex and previously inaccessible anomalies such as superficial CMs, telangiectasias, and deep venous malformations (VMs). When applied continuously, the diode laser effectively acts as a scalpel in ablating highly vascularized defects while keeping the procedure hemostatic; the need for sutures is rarely indicated.[16] Much of the diode laser's popularity among maxillofacial surgeons can be attributed to its modifiable settings, which effectively allow it to carry the function of multiple previously mentioned lasers within a single unit (**Table 1**).

LASER APPLICATION IN VASCULAR ANOMALIES
Capillary Malformations

CMs, also referred to as port-wine-stains, are seen in about 0.5% of infants, presenting at birth and increasing in size during childhood without regression.[17] The presence of CMs during infancy should raise suspicion for a possible congenital sequela; if the V1 dermatome is affected, termed Sturge–Weber, a high suspicion for syndromic involvement should be held and subsequent workup should be initiated. Oftentimes, this is associated with asymmetrical limb hypertrophy (Klippel–Trenaunay) or with acute-onset sensory and motor disturbances (Cobb).

CM pathogenesis relates to the lack of neural innervation to the defective blood vessels within the superficial papillary nexus. This phenomenon results in under activity of sympathetic tone and blood-pooling, ultimately leading to dilation of the vessels. This process is believed to be the foundation of the high posttreatment recurrence rate of CMs. The modern day management of these lesions calls for early action and treatment. If left untouched, the increased size and thickness of the lesion requires high-intensity lasers within a higher number of sessions, placing the individual at more risk of peri- or postoperative complications. Early intervention also improves the social and psychological distress that may precipitate during childhood and beyond.

The argon laser was once the most frequently used in the management of CMs before the advent of PDLs; it delivered an approximately 60% success rate in adults. However, the perioperative pain and high scarring rates in children associated with the argon laser make its use unsuited for the pediatric population. Even in adults, the argon laser's high energy is associated with significant occurrences of hyper- and depigmentation, along with hypertrophic and atrophic scarring.[18] The implementation of the first-generation PDL (577 nm) in CM treatment not only drastically reduced these adverse events in adults but also provided a more effective and suitable option for pediatric cases. The safety and clinical outcomes of PDL use in CM were further improved with the subsequent second-generation PDL (585 nm, 595 nm), which implemented a dynamic cooling device to cool the affected skin in managing perioperative pain. The general PDL parameters for such procedures are set for a 5- to 10-mm spot size and 5 to 8 J/cm^2 energy fluences over a period of 0.45 ms.

Patient expectations should be set early on in the planning for CM laser therapy; current studies report that appropriate clearance of CMs requires on average least 10 laser sessions, with each session being about 2 to 4 weeks apart.[19,20] Treatment time also depends on the patient's Fitzpatrick skin type; increased competing melanin concentration requires both increased treatment sessions and

Table 1
Types of laser and its application in head and neck vascular pathology

Types of Laser	Wavelength	Color	Application in Head and Neck Vascular Pathology
Flash-lamp-pumped pulsed dye laser (PDL)	585 nm, 595 nm	Yellow	Capillary malformations; superficial infantile hemangiomas; telangiectasia
Frequency-doubled Q-switched Nd:YAG (KTP) laser	532 nm	Green	Capillary malformations that are resistant to PDL, such as syndromic CMs that are larger and thicker; telangiectasia; venous malformations
Long-pulsed Nd: YAG laser	1064 nm	Invisible	Capillary malformations that are resistant to PDL, such as syndromic CMs that are deeper, larger, and thicker; telangiectasia; venous malformations
Diode laser	532, 800, 810, 940, and 980 nm	Various	Telangiectasia; venous malformations; excision of highly vascularized lesions such as fibrous hyperplasia

recovery periods to allow for clearance of postoperative pigmentation. Nevertheless, the clinical goal for each procedure is considered complete when either blanching cessation in the targeted area or disappearance of purpura (dark-purplish discoloration) is observed. Although the subtle overlap of the procedure field reduces the development of discoloration with a reticulated pattern, it should be kept at a minimum to reduce damage to surrounding tissues.

CM recurrences of post-laser ablation remain high, with studies reporting a 3% rate of recurrence within 1 year and 40% within 3 years postop.[21] Management of such recurrences is variable, but continued laser treatment can be offered to patients early on when recurrence is first noted and small enough to be managed with short touch-up sessions. Certain CMs that are clinically thick and large, such as those associated with Klippel–Trenaunay syndrome, are more or less resistant to PDL treatment and require the use of other lasers such as the frequency-doubled and long-pulsed 1064-nm Nd:YAG lasers.[22] These lasers function through longer pulse duration, allowing for better accumulation of thermal energy while avoiding vessel rupture in the development of unwarranted purpura.

Infantile Hemangiomas

The efficacy of lasers in the management of infantile hemangiomas (IHs) remains controversial. IHs are a subset of CMs that affect roughly 2.6% of newborns, particularly in 10% of Caucasians.[23] These lesions tend to be absent at birth and subsequently undergo a rapid proliferative phase within the first year. Although 90% are involute by the age 9 years,

these lesions tend to leave long-standing scars and residual tissue remnants.[24] Up to 80% of IHs that do not involute by age of 6 years tend to result in persistent anatomic malformations, although it remains unclear how to adequately predict whether or not a particular lesion will cause future adverse effects.[25] Conventional management of IH consists of monitoring and observing for involution. However, this approach is now losing popularity due to the appreciation for frequent long-term complications of untreated IHs. A common complication of IH sequelae is ulceration which, although relatively benign, may result in numerous psychosocial repercussions for the growing patient. Individualized treatment and managing IHs on a case-by-case basis is therefore necessary to ensure adequate healing with minimal long-term complications.

Recent advances have supported treatment of IHs before the start of the proliferative phase. Treatment in this precursor phase with the PDL specifically has proven to be successful. When the laser is set to 595 nm, 7 J/cm², and 0.150 to 0.300 ms, earlier involution and prevention of deeper vascular infiltration have been observed.[23] Despite this advancement, the benefit of PDL in uncomplicated IH outside of the precursor phase has been unproven. Although propranolol and oral corticosteroids are first-line therapy in the treatment of proliferative phase IH, the PDLs hemostatic, anti-inflammatory, and pain control capabilities are effective in lesions refractory to standard medical management.[26] In vitro studies have shown a significant reduction in vascular endothelial growth factor expression with PDL treatment, pointing to attenuation of key signaling pathways responsible for IH progression.[27] Ablative laser (CO_2, continuous Nd:YAG) may also be used as adjuncts to control IH specifically in the setting of emergent airway compromise.

It is important to note that PDL use is limited to the management of superficial lesions due to its maximal penetration of 1.2 mm. Malformations that lie in deeper tissue must be treated with longer wavelength laser ablation such as with Nd:YAG. The clinician must be mindful of treatment in deeper tissue planes due to postoperative scar formation and dyschromia. Overall, PDL in the management of IH as monotherapy remains controversial. Despite this, the PDL proves to be a promising adjunct to the existing medical therapies (propranolol, timolol maleate 0.5% gel, oral corticosteroids, surgical resection) of IHs, specifically in the ulcerative lesions.[28–30]

Telangiectasia

Telangiectasia is a benign vascular anomaly, in which small vessels (capillaries, venules, arterioles) remain persistently dilated, allowing them to be visible through superficial tissue layers. The PDL has been shown to be an effective treatment modality for maxillofacial telangiectasia due to vessel size (0.1–1.0 mm) and their generally superficial location in the skin. A PDL set to 85 nm, 5 to 7 J/cm^2, and 0.45 ms, in conjunction with cooling devices or cryogen spray allows for efficacious treatment and analgesia. It should be noted that PDL targets overlapping spots of 1.0 mm; appropriate measures should be set in place to avoid significant spot overlap to prevent damage to non-targeted tissue. Excessive spot overlap may result in ulceration, hyperpigmentation, and skin damage. Furthermore, in the setting of spider angioma, in which capillary clusters feed from a larger branching arteriole, all involved vessels must be targeted to prevent recurrence. Clinical success is indicated by eradication of aberrant vessels and formation of light purpura. Focal telangiectasia usually requires one to two treatment sessions for adequate results.[31] Should dark discolorations occur, suspicion should be raised for damage to normal, non-targeted tissue.

Although PDL is effective in treating isolated telangiectasia, it is not generally regarded as curative in the setting of rosacea. Rosacea is a long-term inflammatory condition that causes erythema and rashes of the skin, usually the nasal and malar regions. Recurrence, in this case, is observed to be high due to the disease's chronic inflammatory nature. Pharmacologic management with antibiotics and topical creams may be used for symptomatic disease in certain patients.[32] Telangiectasia associated with rosacea is largely refractive to PDL treatment. Although many avenues have been pursued with medical management, the most effective treatment for rosacea lies in lifestyle modifications.[33]

The most noticeable sequelae of PDL treatment in the setting of telangiectasia is the formation of postoperative purpura. These purpura typically last for up to 2 weeks and tend to be uncomfortable for the patient. Longer PDL (595 nm, 6 to 40 ms, 7 J/cm^2) or KTP lasers may be used for the resolution of postoperative purpura.[4,34,35] The longer pulse duration allows for increased laser energy concentration delivery, which can be titrated to reach the threshold of purpura. Nd:YAG lasers have also been reported to have moderate success rates in the setting of telangiectasia. Isolated telangiectasias have been treated at a rate of 66%, whereas spider angiomas have been cleared with a 93.5% success rate using this modality. The clearance of such lesions is usually reached after one to three sessions.[36] Facial telangiectasias are more receptive to longer PDL therapy than those located elsewhere in the human body. This is likely due to the thin overlying skin layer in the maxillofacial region as compared with other bodily locations. One study demonstrated 75% clearance rates in 93.9% of facial lesions, with the remainder requiring an additional round of laser therapy to acquire the same result.[37] Clinical success with this therapy is identified with vessel blanching or mild erythema. No purpura should be noted with longer PDL treatment. Despite this fact, thicker telangiectasia may still require purpura-induced treatment to allow for clearance.[38]

Venous Malformations

VMs are low-flow vascular anomalies that affect 1 in 10,000 individuals, with roughly 40% occurring in the head and neck region.[39,40] These malformations are present at birth and, in contrast to IH, grow proportionally with the human body. However, certain inciting factors such as puberty, pregnancy, and trauma may result in disproportionate growth of these lesions. Clinically, VMs are soft and take on a purple hue consistent with venous morphology. The Valsalva maneuver may be used to observe for increased flow. A major complication of these low-flow anomalies is the risk of thrombosis due to vascular stasis. Furthermore, VMs are prone to the formation of phleboliths due to calcium deposition, which may result in pain and swelling.[41] Phleboliths may be diagnosed radiographically as hyperdense opacities and may also be mistaken for sialoliths if approximating major/minor salivary glands.

VM treatment is multimodal and dependent on the lesion's size and location. Compression and

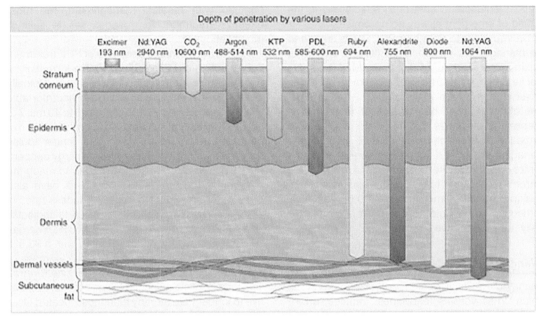

Fig. 2. The laser (indicated in *red*) safely passes through the skin and the heat energy is absorbed by the blood vessels making up the thread vein, breaking down the vessels, and causing them to coagulate. (*From* Tran, H.Q., Manon, V.A., Young, S., Melville, J.C. (2022). Lasers and Nonsurgical Modalities. In: Nair, S.C., Chandra, S.R. (eds) Management of Head and Neck Vascular Lesions. Springer, Singapore. https://doi.org/10.1007/978-981-15-2321-2_10.)

positioning are conservative measures used for lesions in the appendicular region. Sclerotherapy, however, has been a workhorse in the surgical management of VMs in the head and neck. Absolute ethanol (100%) and Ethibloc (alcoholic zein) in addition to Picibanil (OK-432) and Blenoxane (bleomycin) have served as strong sclerotherapeutic agents for VMs. This admixture, however, may result in damage to adjacent structures as well as postoperative fibrosis. Cardiac and renal toxicity has also been observed with the use of such agents.

Laser therapy has developed as an alternative to traditional modalities in treating VM, especially in cases in which the risk of damage to important structures is probable. Owing to the necessity for deep tissue penetration, long wavelength lasers, including Nd:YAG and long diode lasers (810 nm),

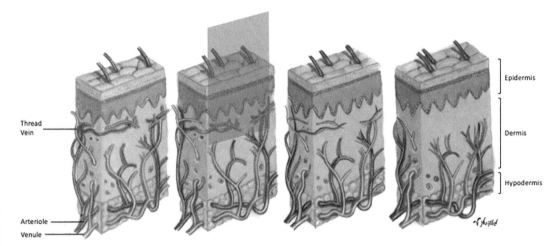

Fig. 3. Effective treatment allows the thread vein to collapse. (*From* Tran, H.Q., Manon, V.A., Young, S., Melville, J.C. (2022). Lasers and Nonsurgical Modalities. In: Nair, S.C., Chandra, S.R. (eds) Management of Head and Neck Vascular Lesions. Springer, Singapore. https://doi.org/10.1007/978-981-15-2321-2_10.)

have been used for head and neck VM treatment. Significant reduction in size of laryngeal VMs and profound improvement of symptoms with Nd:YAG lasers has been reported.[42] Although laser treatment is not always curative, it allows for symptomatic therapy for such lesions. Laser therapy as an adjunct to traditional sclerotherapy or surgical resection limits surgical exposure, allowing for an improved patient experience and more benign postoperative healing period.

SUMMARY

While not devoid of limitations, laser therapy proves to be a promising adjunct to surgical management of vascular anomalies in the head and neck region. Targeted laser therapy allows for healthy tissues to remain intact, thereby promoting superior postoperative site healing as compared with traditional surgical modalities. Continued advancements in laser technology are warranted to improve the practicality of these systems in the clinical setting and allow for its application to more complex and inaccessible pathology. Nevertheless, laser therapy has seen significant progress since its introduction to medical technology and is rapidly gaining more attention and acceptance within maxillofacial surgery. As the clinician's curiosity for adaptation of laser technology continues to prosper, the indications for resulting outcomes of laser therapy in the head and neck region will only continue improving (**Figs. 2** and **3**).

CLINICS CARE POINTS

- Lasers and other nonsurgical modalities should not be considered an all-in-one replacement for surgical measures but instead an adjunct to such traditional approaches to provide more selective and predictable treatment outcomes.

- Maxillofacial surgeons wishing to implement laser therapy should acquire an in-depth understanding and knowledge base of the lasers' mechanisms of action and specific clinical indications before proceeding with such tools in their daily practice.

- Laser technology is a rapidly advancing field and its therapeutic value is consistently improving; as such, practicing surgeons should regularly familiarize themselves with the field's latest advancements and recommendations to offer and deliver the most updated treatment options to their patients.

REFERENCES

1. Geiges ML. History of lasers in dermatology. In: Geiges ML, editor. *Basics in dermatological laser applications*42. Basel, Switzerland: Karger Publishers; 2011. p. 1–6.
2. Waldorf HA, Lask GP, Geronemus RG. Laser treatment of telangiectasias. *Cosm laser surgery*. New York: Wiley and Sons; 1996. p. 71–107.
3. Ng MSY, Tay YK. Laser treatment of infantile hemangiomas. Indian Journal of Paediatric Dermatology 2017;18(3):160.
4. Jasim ZF, Woo WK, Handley JM. Long-pulsed (6-ms) pulsed dye laser treatment of rosacea-associated telangiectasia using subpurpuric clinical threshold. Dermatol Surg 2004;30(1):37–40.
5. Dierickx CC, Casparian JM, Venugopalan V, et al. Thermal relaxation of port-wine stain vessels probed in vivo: the need for 1-10-millisecond laser pulse treatment. J Invest Dermatol 1995;105(5):709–14.
6. Lorenz S, Scherer K, Beatrix Wimmershoff M, et al. Variable pulse frequency-doubled Nd: YAG laser versus flashlamp-pumped pulsed dye laser in the treatment of port wine stains. Acta Derm Venereol 2003;83(3).
7. Clymer MA, Fortune DS, Reinisch L, et al. Interstitial Nd: YAG photocoagulation for vascular malformations and hemangiomas in childhood. Arch Otolaryngol Head Neck Surg 1998;124(4):431–6.
8. Vesnaver A, Dovšak DA. Treatment of large vascular lesions in the orofacial region with the Nd: YAG laser. Journal of cranio-maxillo-facial surgery 2009;37(4):191–5.
9. Civas E, Koc E, Aksoy B, et al. Clinical Experience in the Treatment of Different Vascular Lesions Using a Neodymium-Doped Yttrium Aluminum Garnet Laser. Dermatol Surg 2009;35(12):1933–41.
10. Groot D, Rao J, Johnston P, et al. Algorithm for Using a Long-Pulsed Nd: YAG Laser in the Treatment of Deep Cutaneous Vascular Lesions. Dermatol Surg 2003;29(1):35–42.
11. Yang HY, Zheng LW, Yang HJ, et al. Long-pulsed Nd: YAG laser treatment in vascular lesions of the oral cavity. J Craniofac Surg 2009;20(4):1214–7.
12. Frame JW. Removal of oral soft tissue pathology with the CO2 laser. Journal of oral and maxillofacial surgery 1985;43(11):850–5.
13. Strauss RA, Fallon SD. Lasers in contemporary oral and maxillofacial surgery. Dent Clin North Am 2004;48(4):861–88.
14. Zaffe D, Vitale MC, Martignone A, et al. Morphological, histochemical, and immunocytochemical study of CO2 and Er: YAG laser effect on oral soft tissues. Photomedicine and laser surgery 2004;22(3):185–9.
15. Niamtu J III. The treatment of vascular and pigmented lesions in oral and maxillofacial surgery. Oral Maxillofac Surg Clin 2004;16(2):239–54.

16. Amaral MBF, De Ávila JMS, Abreu MHG, et al. Diode laser surgery versus scalpel surgery in the treatment of fibrous hyperplasia: a randomized clinical trial. Int J Oral Maxillofac Surg 2015;44(11):1383–9.

17. Stratigos AJ, Dover JS, Arndt KA. Laser therapy. Dermatology 2003;2:2153–75.

18. Landthaler M, Hohenleutner U. Laser therapy of vascular lesions. Photodermatol Photoimmunol Photomed 2006;22(6):324–32.

19. Tomson N, Lim SPR, Abdullah A, et al. The treatment of port-wine stains with the pulsed-dye laser at 2-week and 6-week intervals: a comparative study. Br J Dermatol 2006;154(4):676–9.

20. Anolik R, Newlove T, Weiss ET, et al. Investigation into optimal treatment intervals of facial port-wine stains using the pulsed dye laser. J Am Acad Dermatol 2012;67(5):985–90.

21. Orten SS, Waner M, Flock S, et al. Port-wine stains: an assessment of 5 years of treatment. Arch Otolaryngol Head Neck Surg 1996;122(11):1174–9.

22. Savas JA, Ledon JA, Franca K, et al. Pulsed dye laser-resistant port-wine stains: mechanisms of resistance and implications for treatment. Br J Dermatol 2013;168(5):941–53.

23. Stier MF, Glick SA, Hirsch RJ. Laser treatment of pediatric vascular lesions: Port wine stains and hemangiomas. J Am Acad Dermatol 2008;58(2):261–85.

24. Ronchese F. The spontaneous involution of cutaneous vascular tumors. Am J Surg 1953;86(4):376–86.

25. Finn MC, Glowacki J, Mulliken JB. Congenital vascular lesions: clinical application of a new classification. J Pediatr Surg 1983;18(6):894–900.

26. David LR, Malek MM, Argenta LC. Efficacy of pulse dye laser therapy for the treatment of ulcerated haemangiomas: a review of 78 patients. Br J Plast Surg 2003;56(4):317–27.

27. Cao Y, Wang F, Jia Q, et al. One possible mechanism of pulsed dye laser treatment on infantile hemangioma: induction of endothelial apoptosis and serum vascular endothelial growth factor (VEGF) level changes. J Laser Med Sci 2014;5(2):75.

28. Reddy KK, Blei F, Brauer JA, et al. Retrospective study of the treatment of infantile hemangiomas using a combination of propranolol and pulsed dye laser. Dermatol Surg 2013;39(6):923–33.

29. Asilian A, Mokhtari F, Kamali AS, et al. Pulsed dye laser and topical timolol gel versus pulse dye laser in treatment of infantile hemangioma: A double-blind randomized controlled trial. Adv Biomed Res 2015;4.

30. Park KH, Jang YH, Chung HY, et al. Topical timolol maleate 0.5% for infantile hemangioma; it's effectiveness and/or adjunctive pulsed dye laser–single center experience of 102 cases in Korea. J Dermatol Treat 2015;26(4):389–91.

31. Wall TL. Current concepts: laser treatment of adult vascular lesions. Semin Plast Surg 2007;21(No. 3):147. Thieme Medical Publishers.

32. Feldman SR, Huang WW, Huynh TT. Current drug therapies for rosacea: a chronic vascular and inflammatory skin disease. J Manag Care Pharm 2014;20(6):623–9.

33. Weinkle AP, Doktor V, Emer J. Update on the management of rosacea. Clin Cosmet Invest Dermatol 2015;8:159.

34. Tanghetti E, Sherr E. Treatment of telangiectasia using the multi-pass technique with the extended pulse width, pulsed dye laser (Cynosure V-Star). J Cosmet Laser Ther 2003;5(2):71–5.

35. Iyer S, Fitzpatrick RE. Long-pulsed dye laser treatment for facial telangiectasias and erythema: Evaluation of a single purpuric pass versus multiple subpurpuric passes. Dermatol Surg 2005;31(8):898–903.

36. Solak B, Sevimli Dikicier B, Oztas Kara R, et al. Single-center experience with potassium titanyl phosphate (KTP) laser for superficial cutaneous vascular lesions in face. J Cosmet Laser Ther 2016;18(8):428–31.

37. Cassuto DA, Ancona DM, Emanuelli G. Treatment of facial telangiectasias with a diode-pumped Nd: YAG Laser at 532nm. J Cutan Laser Ther 2000;2(3):141–6.

38. Alam M, Dover JS, Arndt KA. Treatment of facial telangiectasia with variable-pulse high-fluence pulsed-dye laser: Comparison of efficacy with fluences immediately above and below the purpura threshold. Dermatol Surg 2003;29(7):681–5.

39. Boon LM, Mulliken JB, Enjolras O, et al. Glomuvenous malformation (glomangioma) and venous malformation: distinct clinicopathologic and genetic entities. Arch Dermatol 2004;140(8):971–6.

40. Mulliken JB, Fishman SJ, Burrows PE. Vascular anomalies. Curr Probl Surg 2000;37(8):517–84.

41. Scolozzi P, Laurent F, Lombardi T, et al. Intraoral venous malformation presenting with multiple phleboliths. Oral Surg Oral Med Oral Pathol Oral Radiol Endod 2003;96(2):197–200.

42. Glade R, Vinson K, Richter G, et al. Endoscopic management of airway venous malformations with Nd: YAG laser. Ann Otol Rhinol Laryngol 2010;119(5):289–93.

Indications, Options, and Updates on Embolic Agents

Jesse G.A. Jones, MD

KEYWORDS

• Embolization • Sclerotherapy • High flow • Low flow • Percutaneous

KEY POINTS

- Define the role of intervention with respect to an overall treatment goal.
- Use an interventional technique suited to the class of vascular anomaly.
- Manage patient and family expectations at the outset.

INTRODUCTION

Vascular anomalies (VAs) of the head and neck are diverse in terms of flow state, size, and location.[1,2] These factors influence a given VA's symptomatology, functional and psychosocial impact. When treatment is indicated, the role of intervention must first be defined as either sole therapy with curative or palliative intent or adjunctive to surgery and/or medication. Interventional strategy itself is dictated by lesion characteristics, most importantly the flow state. Low-flow lymphatic or venous VAs are primarily treated by percutaneous sclerotherapy,[3] whereas catheter-directed embolization applies more to high-flow arterial or arteriovenous VAs (**Table 1**). Nevertheless, VAs represent a continuous spectrum, and so the treatment approach similarly demonstrates some degree of overlap.

INDICATIONS/CONTRAINDICATIONS

Intervention in VAs aims for fluid (lymph and/or blood) reduction and is, therefore, directed toward the cellular lining of each lesion. VAs composed primarily of avascular stromal components are ill-suited targets. Similarly, reactive changes in adjacent tissue such as bony hypertrophy in high-flow VAs or scarring from repeated hemorrhage are not addressed by flow cessation alone. The ideal agent balances efficacy with safety, whereas sclerosing liquids such as absolute ethanol potently denude vascular endothelium and penetrate deeply; these same properties expose healthy tissue to significant risk from untoward embolization when highly selective exposure is not achieved. A sclerosant's efficacy depends not only on its intrinsic mechanism of action but also on variables such as concentration and dwell time.

TECHNIQUE/PROCEDURE

Preoperative Planning

One must first complete a thorough history, physical examination, and review of the imaging. VA's wax and wane alongside trauma, inflammation, and infection. Performing a brief bedside ultrasound may reveal marked involution and prompt one to cancel treatment before anesthetic induction, draping, and opening of sterile instruments and agents.

For VAs adjacent to the airway, an extubation plan should be formulated in advance with the anesthesia and otolaryngology teams; patients at high risk of asphyxiation from postoperative edema remain intubated overnight or may even require tracheostomy if multistaged treatments are planned. Some agents, such as bleomycin, require specific advance contact precautions to prevent skin discoloration (see **Table 1**). An

University of Alabama at Birmingham, FOT 1007, 1720 2nd Avenue South, Birmingham, AL 35294-3410, USA
E-mail address: jessejones@uabmc.edu

Oral Maxillofacial Surg Clin N Am 36 (2024) 29–34
https://doi.org/10.1016/j.coms.2023.09.006
1042-3699/24/

Table 1
Embolic agents

Agent	Mechanism of Action	Adverse Reactions	Notes
EVOH	Ethylene vinyl polymerizes into a solid cast as dimethyl sulfoxide (DMSO) solvent diffuses away	DMSO causes vascular necrosis in high concentrations; infuse at 0.1 mL/10 s	Patient emits foul odor as DMSO diffuses out of the body. Do not exceed 1.5 mL/kg EVOH per session
N-BCA glue[12]	Cyanoacrylate polymerizes in ionic medium such as blood	Polymerization time cannot be precisely determined a priori. Therefore, nontarget embolization may occlude flow in undesired locations	Several factors affect n-BCA polymerization including ethiodized oil dilution, vessel flow, diameter, and tortuosity. Skilled use requires experience
PVA	Plastic beads travel with flowing blood until the vessel tapers and the particle lodges into an occlusive position	Small particles (<250 µm) penetrate deeper into the vascular bed and may result in ischemic necrosis of skin, nerve, or other tissues if off-target embolization occurs	Must be injected under conditions of free flow to prevent pressurization of the pedicle and subsequent passage of PVA though unseen anastomoses
Ethanol	Fibrinoid necrosis via protein denaturation, desiccation, and thrombosis	• Cardiopulmonary collapse (systemic infusion, eg, high-flow VA) • Tissue necrosis[a] in off-target embolization	Recommended dosage is 1 mL/kg or less. In high-flow VA, do not exceed 0.14 mL/kg/bolus and wait 10 min between bolus injections
Polidocanol[13]	Endothelial cell death via calcium signaling and nitric oxide pathways	• Cerebral or pulmonary air embolism if foamed sclerosant passes through dangerous anastomoses[b]	Most data on use are from venous sclerotherapy although telangiectasia has also been successfully treated
Sodium tetradecyl sulfate (STS)[14]	Detergent action dissolves lipids composing endothelial cell membrane	• Cerebral or pulmonary air embolism if foamed sclerosant passes through dangerous anastomoses[b]	Commonly used agent due to favorable side effect profile and efficacy, especially when foamed
Doxycycline	Inflammation, matrix metalloproteinase, and VEGF inhibition	Tissue necrosis in off-target embolization	Inexpensive. Commonly used in microcystic low-flow VA
Bleomycin[15]	DNA degradation through inhibition of thymidine incorporation	• Pulmonary fibrosis at high doses (has been reported with chemo-therapy but not sclerotherapy use) • Skin discoloration at site of adhesives and prolonged pressure if left in place during infusion and/or removed before 24 h	Recommended dosage is 0.5 IU/kg per procedure, not exceeding 15 IU. Lifetime maximum of 400 IU

(continued on next page)

Table 1 (continued)			
Agent	**Mechanism of Action**	**Adverse Reactions**	**Notes**
OK-432	Stimulation of host immunity	• Regional inflammatory response may be exuberant and if involving the airway, can lead to dyspnea[c] • Intralesional hemorrhage[c]	Successful trial in LM completed in 2007[16] but FDA approval lapsed. Further trials are currently ongoing to reintroduce agent into US market

[a] Although all sclerosants may cause tissue necrosis if extravasation outside the confines of a VA occurs, ethanol tends to be the most severe.

[b] Air embolism is a risk with any foamed sclerosant, the most common agents being STS and polidocanol. Venous use predisposes to pulmonary emboli, whereas arterial (eg, telangiectasia) use in the head and neck predisposes to cerebral emboli.

[c] Reported in numerous other sclerosing agents.

Abbreviations: FDA, food and drug administration; LM, lymphatic malformation; VEGF, vascular endothelial growth factor.

anesthetic plan for awake patients must also be determined if general anesthesia is not used. Sparse medical evidence supports prophylactic antibiotic use, although the practice is commonplace and directed toward skin and/or oral flora, depending on the planned access.[4–6]

Prep and Patient Positioning

Ready access to the VA and adequate visualization during treatment are of paramount importance. Let the lesion location determine supine, prone, or decubitus positioning. Oral VAs may benefit from nasal intubation and dental bite blocks. Performing ultrasound and/or fluoroscopy before prepping and draping may inform changes in positioning such as flexion or extension, use of towel rolls or "bumps" that optimize access and image quality.

Surgical Approach

International society for the study of vascular anomalies (ISSVA) class and treatment goal (adjunct vs sole therapy) strongly influence interventional strategy. Specific paradigms indexed by VA type are described below, yet the principles dictating safe and effective therapy are uniform. Many agents are toxic, and even inert substances like polyvinyl alcohol (PVA) may be harmful if deposited into eloquent tissue. Therefore, all embolization must be confined as much as feasible to the VA itself and treatment withheld if highly targeted delivery cannot be ensured. Live visual feedback through fluoroscopy and/or ultrasound is performed during infusion to monitor distribution within the VA.

High-flow arteriovenous malformations (AVMs) and fistulas (AVFs) pose risk of significant intraoperative blood loss, and therefore, the interventional approach focuses on flow reduction. Transarterial, venous, or direct puncture approaches are informed by prior cross-sectional imaging such as computed tomography (CT) or MR angiography and ultrasound. Adjunct treatment provides more latitude among embolic agents: although particles are often transiently effective, they last the days leading up to surgery. Permanent embolics such as coils, N-butyl cyanoacrylate (n-BCA), and ethylene vinyl alcohol (EVOH), however, may leave a noncosmetic mass or black discoloration (from tantalum) but these can be removed during resection. Intervention should target the venous recipient of the arteriovenous shunt. Outlet thrombosis triggers involution of the entire VA, as proangiogenic molecular signaling ceases.[7] Alternatively, perivascular bleomycin infusion has been recently described as a means involuting AVMs by triggering endothelial apoptosis.[8]

Capillary malformations such as hemangioma contain arterial feeding pedicles but demonstrate less rapid flow by the virtue of a microvascular network between artery and vein. Transarterial embolization with polymer-based particles such PVA exploits this network by depositing 150 to 300 μm beads. Liquid embolics may also be used to close the feeding artery and penetrate into the capillary bed. As with AVMs, perivascular bleomycin (with or without triamcinolone) infusion has also been described.[9]

Venous malformations (VMs) typically flow slowly enough that a liquid-based sclerotherapy agent has sufficient dwell time to denude the local vascular endothelium before washing out. The smallest caliber microcystic VMs exhibit fragile vascular channels (<500 μm) with sufficiently slow flow to warrant a gravity drip technique using a pure liquid agent.[10] However, most others benefit from additional flow control techniques to maximize dwell time and reduce systemic concentration of these toxic agents. Sclerosant viscosity may be increased by mixing with gelfoam, avatine and/or air to create a slurry; needles of at least 20 G should be used to prevent blockage. Applying a tourniquet, manual compression, or even coiling off the draining vein(s) represent additional strategies.

Lymphatic malformations (LMs) are the slowest flowing VAs and may be considered stagnant for practical purposes. Dilution, rather than washout, poses a challenge to treatment efficacy. Remove as much lymphatic fluid as possible before instilling sclerosant either by gravity or aspiration (through an 18 G or larger needle), depending on viscosity. Techniques for optimizing surface area contact include foaming sclerosants with air and/or Gelfoam as well as infusing one agent such as sodium tetradecyl for 10 to 15 minutes then aspirating and infusing a second such as doxycycline[11] (**Figs. 1** and **2**).

Postoperative Care

Once the needle is removed, manual compression is applied to prevent bleeding or leakage of the embolic agent. A sterile dressing is applied, except in the case of bleomycin because adhesives may impart skin discoloration if removed within 24 hours. Patients and families are counseled to expect mild-to-moderate pain and swelling locally and may use non-steroidal anti-inflammatory drugs (NSAIDs) and acetaminophen as needed. Patients whose VA is located adjacent to the aerodigestive tract warrant particular vigilance because postoperative edema poses risk of asphyxiation. Allow 4 to 6 weeks between clinic follow-up for embolization to demonstrate its full effect. Additional sessions may be indicated if response is incomplete or unsatisfactory.

Possible Complications and Management

Sclerosant extravasation into adjacent tissues will result in a pronounced inflammatory response characterized by pain, swelling as well as potential skin necrosis, and loss of function from peripheral nerve injury or mass effect. Mild injuries can be managed conservatively, whereas more serious adverse events require directed intervention from specialists on an urgent basis. Hyperpigmentation associated with bleomycin fades with time but may not completely resolve.[11–18] Additional agent-specific information can be found in **Table 1**.

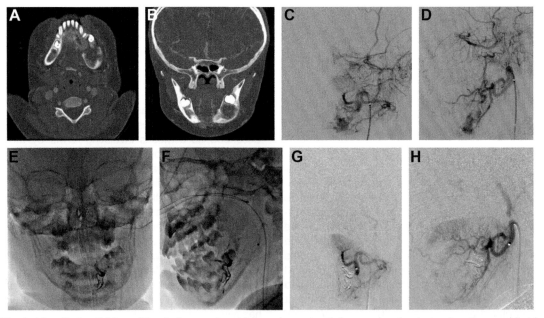

Fig. 1. Mandibular AVM resulting in frequent oral hemorrhage, tooth loss, and malocclusion in a 2-year-old girl. Otherwise healthy. CT angiogram in axial (A) and coronal (B) planes demonstrates a nidal structure in the floor of mouth and ectatic draining vein remodeling and expanding the mandible. Left external carotid artery (ECA) digital subtraction angiogram in frontal (C) and lateral (D) planes depicts the vasculature in detail. A mental branch of the facial artery supplies the AVM and represents a target for embolization. Radiographs of subsequent EVOH cast (frontal E; lateral F). Postembolization left ECA angiogram shows no residual AVM filling from this pedicle (frontal G; lateral H). The patient subsequently underwent extraction of a right mandibular molar tooth and excision of adjacent pyogenic granuloma with minimal blood loss.

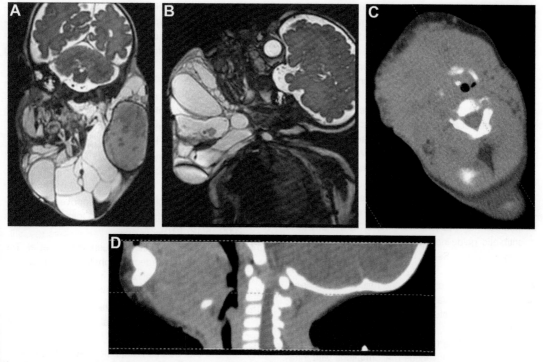

Fig. 2. An 18-month-old boy who underwent intubation following caesarian section for an extensive facial lymphatic malformation (MRI Face in coronal *A* and sagittal *B* planes). He subsequently underwent surgical de-bulking, yet encountered difficulty weaning off tracheostomy and G-tube. Residual epiglottic VA was implicated on endoscopy. Intralesional bleomycin was injected percutaneously, under CT guidance (axial *C* depicts needle tip anterior to the trachea; sagittal reconstruction of scout image before needle insertion with pink reference *line* for comparison *D*). The tracheostomy and G-tube were eventually removed.

SUMMARY

Embolic agents represent a diverse class of minimally invasive therapies for a wide range of VAs. They are useful either as surgical adjuncts or as monotherapy. When crafting a treatment plan, it is essential to consider not only the type of VA, that is, high or low flow but also the long-term goals, understanding that complete removal often comes with unacceptable morbidity.

CLINICS CARE POINTS

- When treating lesions adjacent to the aerodigestive tract, consider periprocedural corticosteroids to reduce swelling. Prepare for airway compromise by using nebulizers, overnight hospital admission, and prolonged intubation/endotracheal (ET) tube leak testing as needed.
- In lesions with brisk washout such as some venous malformations and any arteriovenous (AV) shunt, a flow control strategy such as manual compression, intravenous balloon occlusion, or coiling is needed to ensure adequate dwell time and prevent systemic accumulation of the sclerosant.
- Sclerosant injections should be monitored in real time using either fluoroscopy (if admixed with iodinated contrast) or ultrasound to ensure intralesional deposition with no or minimal extravasation into healthy adjacent tissues.

DISCLOSURE

Consultant for Cerenovus, a supplier of N-BCA glue.

Consultant and medical advisory board member for Protara, a supplier of OK-432.

REFERENCES

1. ISSVA Classification Available at: https://www.issva.org/classification. Accessed date 09 March 2023.
2. Kunimoto K, Yamamoto Y, Jinnin M. ISSVA classification of vascular anomalies and molecular biology. Int J Mol Sci 2022;23(4).

3. De Maria L, De Sanctis P, Balakrishnan K, et al. Sclerotherapy for venous malformations of head and neck: systematic review and meta-analysis. Neurointervention 2020;15(1):4–17.

4. Pimpalwar S. Vascular malformations: approach by an interventional radiologist. Semin Plast Surg 2014;28(2):91–103.

5. Chehab MA, Thakor AS, Tulin-Silver S, et al. Adult and pediatric antibiotic prophylaxis during vascular and ir procedures: a society of interventional radiology practice parameter update endorsed by the cardiovascular and interventional radiological society of europe and the canadian association for interventional radiology. J Vasc Intervent Radiol 2018; 29(11):1483–14501 e2.

6. Moon E, Tam MD, Kikano RN, et al. Prophylactic antibiotic guidelines in modern interventional radiology practice. Semin Intervent Radiol 2010;27(4): 327–37.

7. Mullan S. Reflections upon the nature and management of intracranial and intraspinal vascular malformations and fistulae. J Neurosurg 1994;80(4): 606–16.

8. Jin Y, Zou Y, Hua C, et al. Treatment of Early-stage extracranial arteriovenous malformations with intralesional interstitial bleomycin injection: a pilot study. Radiology 2018;287(1):194–204.

9. Tiwari P, Bera RN, Pandey V. Bleomycin-triamcinolone sclerotherapy in the management of propranolol resistant infantile hemangioma of the maxillofacial region: A single arm prospective evaluation of clinical outcome and Doppler ultrasound parameters. J Stomatol Oral Maxillofac Surg 2023;124(1S): 101313.

10. Berenstein A, Bazil MJ, Sorscher M, et al. Percutaneous sclerotherapy of microcystic lymphatic malformations: the use of an innovative gravity-dependent technique. J Neurointerventional Surg 2023;15(3):272–5.

11. Caton MT, Baker A, Smith ER, et al. Dual-agent percutaneous sclerotherapy technique for macrocystic lymphatic malformations. J Neurointerventional Surg 2022. https://doi.org/10.1136/jnis-2022-019255.

12. Hill H, Chick JFB, Hage A, et al. N-butyl cyanoacrylate embolotherapy: techniques, complications, and management. Diagn Interv Radiol 2018;24(2): 98–103.

13. Eckmann DM. Polidocanol for endovenous microfoam sclerosant therapy. Expet Opin Invest Drugs 2009;18(12):1919–27.

14. Alakailly X, Kummoona R, Quereshy FA, et al. The use of sodium tetradecyl sulphate for the treatment of venous malformations of the head and neck. J Maxillofac Oral Surg 2015;14(2):332–8.

15. Cheng J. Doxycycline sclerotherapy in children with head and neck lymphatic malformations. J Pediatr Surg 2015;50(12):2143–6.

16. Giguere CM, Bauman NM, Sato Y, et al. Treatment of lymphangiomas with OK-432 (Picibanil) sclerotherapy: a prospective multi-institutional trial. Arch Otolaryngol Head Neck Surg 2002;128(10):1137–44.

17. Albanese G, Kondo KL. Pharmacology of sclerotherapy. Semin Intervent Radiol 2010;27(4):391–9.

18. Milbar HC, Jeon H, Ward MA, et al. Hyperpigmentation after foamed bleomycin sclerotherapy for vascular malformations. J Vasc Intervent Radiol 2019;30(9):1438–42.

Terminology and Classifications of Vascular Lesions Based on Molecular Identification

Srinivasa R. Chandra, MD, BDS, FDS, FIBCSOMS[a],*, Advaith Nair, MBBS[a],
Sanjiv Nair, MDS, FFDRCS, FDSRCPS, FIBSCOMS[b]

KEYWORDS

- Vascular lesion • Hemangioma • Vascular malformation • Lymphangioma

KEY POINTS

- No single susceptible population group has been identified. So classifications and historical understanding of vascular lesions is critical, to know the self-limiting versus aggressive lesions, typical clinical appearance etc.
- When surgical or interventional therapy is contemplated, need-based imaging studies play a major role.
- Majority are benign entities and not "cancers". Conservative management versus resection for lesion eradication *should not be a piecemeal* methodology.
- There is no *one* treatment modality which would fit every vascular anomaly.
- Biopsy of the lesions may not be necessary; *malformations are more common*. Biopsy only if you understand it has malignant behavior.
- Vascular anomalies have a "*dynamic lifecycle*". Biological syndrome-based grouping was logistical convenience, but with mutational foundations, the syndromes are reclassified.
- Between vascular tumors and malformations, tumors are more common, but you may encounter 'malformation' more often as they persist and need varied care. Patients usually present with multiple earlier investigations and interventions.
- Vascular anomalies—'group' of different entities of varied etio-pathological which may not share same treatments approaches.
- Airway/vision must be a consideration in managing head and neck anomalies, especially with syndromes and segmental presentations.
- Great potential for molecular and genetic research in this field-so multispecialty clinics save tissue samples for research laboratories for discovering targeted therapies.

INTRODUCTION

This article may provide a comprehensive understanding of vascular-related entities and updates on classifications.

Majority of the vascular anomalies are seen in the head and neck region. Even though the incidence of this anomaly could be construed as a rare disease entity, with only 5% of overall affliction, the lack of knowledgeable management has disfigured many. A comprehensive understanding of this benign yet complex life-changing entity is essential. A historical perspective, pathophysiology-logical evolution, and the current knowledge of management

[a] Department of Oral and Maxillofacial Surgery - Head and Neck Oncology and Microvascular Reconstruction, Oregon Health and Sciences University, 3181 SW Sam Jackson Park Road, Portland, OR 97239, USA; [b] B M Jain Hospital, Bangalore Institute of Dental Sciences, 35, 4th Main 13 Cross, Malleswaram, Bangalore, 560003
* Corresponding author
E-mail address: chandrsr@ohsu.edu

Oral Maxillofacial Surg Clin N Am 36 (2024) 35–48
https://doi.org/10.1016/j.coms.2023.09.010

modalities are essential for rendering clinical care in this subspecialty care.

HISTORY

The first scientifically documented "surgery under an ether anesthetic agent" by Morton in 1846 done in Boston, Massachusetts, USA, was for excision of a "low-flow" vascular malformation. Rudolph Virchow, in 1863, first categorized vascular anomalies by microscopic architectural patterns. From earlier use words "port wine stain," "angiomas," etc. Virchow attempted an acceptable cellular classification as angioma simplex, angioma cavernosum, and angioma rac-emosum. The further biological classification was proposed in 1982 by Mulliken and Glowacki.[1] The international collaborative group—International Society for the Study of Vascular Anomalies (ISSVA)—is a way forward to advance constant review of the current and updated science in this field.[2]

Classifications for vascular lesions are complex. Vascular tumors have increased mitotic activity and will appear soon after birth, with approximately 30% already apparent at the time of birth.[1,3] Vascular tumors are divided by the ISSVA as benign, locally aggressive or borderline, and malignant. Benign tumors include hemangiomas. Locally aggressive or borderline tumors include Kaposi Sarcoma and hemangioendothelioma. Malignant tumors include angiosarcomas and epithelioid hemangioendothelioma (**Table 1**).

INCIDENCE

The overall incidence of vascular lesions is around 5%.[4] Among tumors, infantile hemangiomas have the same percentage of incidence. Among vascular lesions, venous malformations are commonly like lymphatic malformations with an incidence of 1:5000 to 1:10000.

More than 50% of them are present in the head and neck anatomic area.[2]

TERMINOLOGY AND CLASSIFICATIONS

Terminology of vascular lesions evolved from descriptive to the more scientific basis for nomenclature, the former possibly arising from maternal explanations of the lesions. It posted 1982 after Mulliken and Glowacki and colleagues[1] attributed biologic differences within the lesion that they were described as separate entities. A neoplastic hemangioma was found to be distinctly different from the developmental vascular malformation.

Historical Terminology on Appearances

Descriptive terms and historical nosology of vascular anomalies offer an array of overlapping descriptive and histopathologic terms.

Port wine can be used for "capillary hemangiomas" historically. It can be as small and superficial.

Histopathologic terms used historically

- Capillary

Table 1
Various classification of vascular anomalies

Year	Author	Basis of classification
1863	Virchow RLK	Microscopic channel architecture
1877	Wegener	Histomorphic subclassification of Virchow's classification
1973	Degni and coworkers	Site of origin of the detect
1974	Malan	Embryologic site of origin of the defect
1982	Mulliken JB and Glowacki J	Endothelial characters
1983	Burrows and colleagues	Angiographic flow patterns
1988	International Society for the Study of Vascular Anomalies (ISSVA), Hamburg	Anatomopathologic classification of vascular defects (Hamburg classification)
1989	Belov	Etiologic and pathophusiologic classification system
1992	ISSVA, Colorado	Cellular features, vascular flow, characteristics and clonincal behavior
1993	Jackson and associates	Flow rate
1996	ISSVA, Rome	Modified ISSVA classification
2011	S C Nair	Anatomical presentation
2014	ISSVA, Melbourne	Modified ISSVA classification

Adopted from Nair, Chandra Management of Head and Neck Vascular Lesions: A Guide for Surgeons, Springer Nature, Edition 1, May 2022; https://doi.org/10.1007/978-981-15-2321-2; ISBN978-981-15-2320-5.

Box 1
Vascular anomalies Classification system.

International society for the study of vascular Anomalies classification system (ISSVA, last revision 2022, please review at ISSVA.org)

Vascular tumors

  Benign

  Locally aggressive or borderline

  Malignant

Vascular malformations

  Simple

    Capillary malformations

    Lymphatic malformations

    Venous malformations

    Arteriovenous malformations

    Arteriovenous fistula

  Combined (2 or more VMs in one lesion)

    CVM, CLM, LVM, CLVM, CAVM, CLAVM, others

- Cavernous
- Arterial
- Mixed

Strawberry lesion or a "capillary-cavernous hemangioma" was commonly used for lesions like present on the tongue. Such terminology added to the confusion as shown in a tongue vascular lesion, which is a low-flow vascular lesion, with sequela of trauma.

MULLIKEN AND GLOWACKI'S BIOLOGICAL CLASSIFICATION (1982)

The ISSVA classification has been modified and based on the biologic classification by Mulliken and Glowacki[1] and further with the mutational knowledge (**Box 1** and **Fig. 1**).

Hemangiomas

Proliferating phase

- Involuting phase.

Malformations

- Capillary
- Venous
- Arterial
- Lymphatic
- Fistulas
- Hemangioma

Further advances in the understanding of the vascular dynamics allowed changes in the classification, and this was first proposed by Ian Jackson and colleagues, allowing major breakthroughs in treatment planning and management of vascular lesions.

M.Ethunandan et al., [5] bjoms 44(2006) described a flow chart that correlated the various clinical signs, which helped differentiate a Vascular malformation from a Hemangioma.

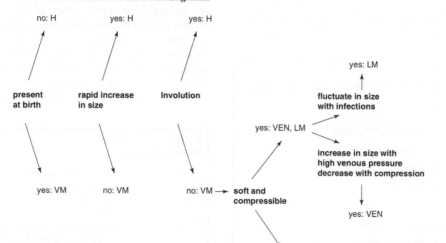

Fig. 1. Described a flow chart that correlated the various clinical signs, which helped differentiate a Vascular malformation from a Hemangioma, arterial malformation-AM; AV, fistula; AVM, arteriovenous malformation; AVH, hemangioma; VM, vascular malforma-tion; LM, lym-phatic malformation; VEN, venous malformation. (*From* M.Ethunandan and colleagues,[5] bjoms 44(2006))

Box 2
Classification of non-CNS vascular malformations.

Haemangiomas (proliferative lesions or tumors)

Vascular malformations (non-proliferative)

High flow

- Arteriovenous malformations

Low flow:

- Capillary malformations
- Venous malformations
- Lymphatic malformations
- Mixed malformations

From: Management of Head and Neck Vascular Lesions: A Guide for Surgeons, Springer Nature, Edition 1, May 2022; https://doi.org/10.1007/978-981-15-2321-2; ISBN978-981-15-2320-5.

CENTRAL NERVOUS SYSTEM AND NON-CENTRAL NERVOUS SYSTEM LIST OF VASCULAR LESIONS

Central nervous system vascular malformations are rare abnormalities of blood vessels in your brain or spinal cord and their membranes. They distinctly differ in their appearance and management (**Boxes 2–5** and **Table 2**).[2]

PATHOGENESIS

Blood vessels form consolidated aberrations in limited anatomic sites of the human body. They result in sporadic anomalies or hereditary occurrences. Hemangiomas are vascular neoplasms that have different phases of development. They

Box 3
Classification of CNS vascular malformations

Arteriovenous shunts

Classical AV Malformations

Pial AV fistulas

Dural AV shunts

Galenic shunts

Cavernous malformations

Capillary telangiectasias

Venous malformations

Developmental venous

Anomalies

Mixed malformations

Box 4
Classified both Hemangiomas and VM based on their anatomic location.

IAN JACKSON IN 1992 further expanded on the earlier classification. Based on this, Hemangiomas were described on their location and VM on the dynamixs of blood flow.

Hemangiomas

Superficial (capillary hemangioma)

Deep (cavernous hemangioma)

Compound (capillary-cavernous hemangioma)

Vascular malformations

Simple lesions

Low flow lesions

Capillary malformations (capillary hemangioma, port wine satin)

Venous malformation (cavernous hemangioma)

Lymphatic malformation (lymphangioma, cystic hygroma)

High-flow lesions

Arterial malformation

Combine lesions

Arteriovenous malformations

Lymph venous malformations

Other combinations

From: More recently Sanjiv Nair and colleagues[4]

go through the proliferative phase, quiescent phase, and finally involutory phase. Histologically they are characterized by the proliferation of plump endothelial cells with mast cell infiltration.[5,6] Infantile hemangiomas show increased expression of glucose transporter-1. The cellular activity during involution shows the reduction in angiogenesis

Box 5
Based on Types

Type I	Mucosal/cultaneous
Type II	Subcutaneous/juxta muscular
Type III	Glandular
Type IV	Skeletal (intra bony)
Type V	Deep visceral (temporal, infra temporal, parapharyngeal)

Adopted from Nair, Chandra Management of Head and Neck Vascular Lesions: A Guide for Surgeons, Springer Nature, Edition 1, May 2022; https://doi.org/10.1007/978-981-15-2321-2; ISBN978-981-15-2320-5.

Table 2
Schobinger Classification: Schobinger clinical staging system of arteriovenous malformations

Stage I	Quiescence	Cutaneous blush, skin warmth, arteriovenous shunt on doppler Ultrasound
Stage II	Expansion	Darkening blush, lesion shows pulsation, thrill and bruit
Stage III	Destruction	Steal, distal ischemia, pain, dystrophic skin changes, ulceration, necrosis, soft tissue and bony changes
Stage IV	Decompensation	High-output cardiac failure

As adopted from Schobinger's classification: Adopted from Nair, Chandra Management of Head and Neck Vascular Lesions: A Guide for Surgeons, Springer Nature, Edition 1, May 2022; https://doi.org/10.1007/978-981-15-2321-2; ISBN978-981-15-2320-5.

with apoptosis of endothelial cells. Congenital hemangiomas in contrast are fully mature at birth and do not show a proliferative phase. Pathogenesis is a complex interaction of genetic and environmental factors. The role of human papillomavirus-8 infection, chronic villus sampling, and hormonal, especially estrogen disturbances with possible hypoxia causing endothelial cell proliferation is another theory.[4–6] The role and efficacy of beta 2 blockers in the management of proliferating hemangiomas are documented.[7–9] Vascular malformations are the result of errors in angiogenesis. The growth and differentiation of vascular lesion and endothelium are driven by 2 major pathways: RAS/RAF and PIK3CA (Refer to **Fig. 2**).[2]

vascular endothelial growth factor (VEGF) and platelet-derived growth factor, growth factors of Raf, Ras in tyrosine class receptors Ras and Raf are downstream from the 2-peptide amino acid class tyrosine kinase, which is the first step receptor in cancer and vascular cell upregulation.[2]

G Protein-related spectrum: There are multiple G protein receptors related mutations on genes of GNA Q/GNA 11/GNA 14.[10,11] A few instances of this GNA vascular anomaly spectrum anomalies are congenital hemangioma, capillary hemangioma, kaposiform hemangioendothelioma.

PIK3CA-related overgrowth spectrum (PROS):[11–16] Vascular anomalies caused by PIK3CA related mutations are known as PROS. The majority of the known vascular anomalies' mutations are associated with the tyrosine kinase receptor-associated signaling pathway of RAS and PIK3CA.

Mutations and Vascular Lesions

Mutations can be of 2 broad types: Germline and Somatic (**Box 6**).

THERAPEUTIC HYPOTHESES

For the treatment of vascular diseases[2,17–23] (**Fig. 3**)

Pathogenesis

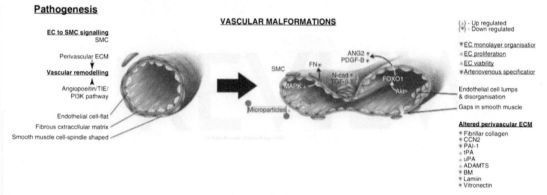

Fig. 2. Normal vascular lumen lined with endothelial cells with normal radiation, surrounding fibrosis extracellular matrix, and spindle-shaped smooth muscle cell layer. SMC Smooth muscle cell, EC Endothelial cell, ECM Extracellular matrix; Somatic mutations causing 'gain of function' in the tyrosine kinase receptor of -ANG (Angiopoietin) type, TIE and PIK3CA encoding genes activated cell signaling pathway leading to vascular malformations. In experimental mouse models of angiogene-sis ANG/TIE/PIK3CA cause cell signaling and perivascular extracellular matrix remodeling, degradation, etc. (*Adapted from* Kangas J, Nätynki M, Eklund L. Development of Molecular Therapies for Venous Malformations. Basic Clin Pharmacol Toxicol. 2018 Sep;123 Suppl 5:6–19. https://doi.org/10.1111/ bcpt.13027. Epub 2018 May 29. PMID: 29668117.All right reserved to Brishank Pratop © 2021.)

Targeting the PI3K/AKT/mTOR Pathway

- Mammalian target for rapamycin (mTOR) inhibitors, such as rapamycin in vascular malformation, multiple cutaneous and mucosal venous malformation, mixed vascular malformation, blue rubber bleb nervous, and lymphatic malformation; also hereditary hemorrhagic telangiectasia (HHT)? Targeting the RAS/BRAF/MAPK/ERK pathway
- Possible inhibitors could be the BRAF inhibitor vemurafenib or the mitogen activating pathway kinase-extracellular signal-regulated kinase (MEK) inhibitor trametinib.in capillary malformation (CM), CM-arteriovenous malformation 1 (CM-AVM1) and CM-AVM2, pyogenic granuloma (PG), noninvoluting congenital hemangioma (NICH), rapidly involuting congenital hemangioma (RICH), and verrucous venous malformations. Targeting angiogenesis
- Antiangiogenic agents, such as bevacizumab in HHT, IH.

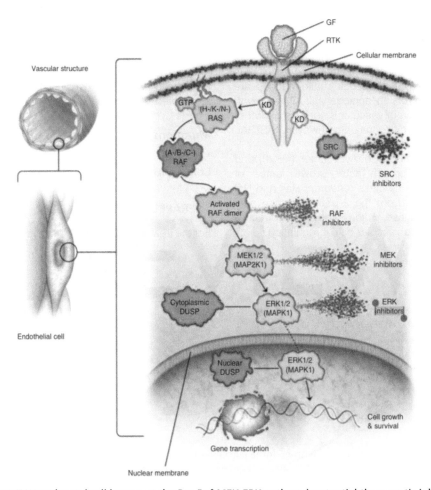

Fig. 3. MAPK/ERK pathway (well known as the Ras-Raf-MEK-ERK pathway) potential therapeutic inhibitors. Protein chain in a vascular cell that transmits signal from a cell surface receptor to the DNA in the cell nucleus. (*Adopted from* Nair, Chandra Management of Head and Neck Vascular Lesions: A Guide for Surgeons, Springer Nature, Edition 1, May 2022; https://doi.org/10.1007/978-981-15-2321-2; ISBN978–981–15–2320–5.). (All right reserved to Brishank Pratop © 2021.)

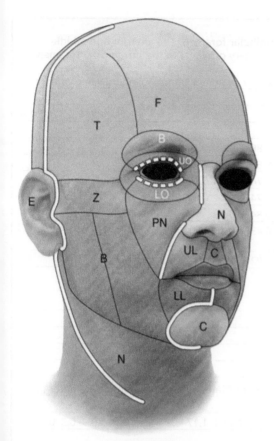

Fig. 4. Facial incisions based on aesthetic subunits. (All right reserved to Brishank Pratop © 2021.)

- Targeting transforming growth factor (TGF)-ß pathway
- Glomuvenous malformation (GVM)

Growth and differentiation of the vascular lesion and its endothelial cell proliferation or initiated at the cell membrane tyrosine kinase receptor with the RAS- RAF downstream to nucleus MAPK dependent gene transcription. The illustration **Fig. 3** demonstrates the potential therapy and inhibition of Src-tyrosine kinase family.Inhibitors; rapidly accelerated fibrosarcoma (RAF) inhibitors; mitogen activating pathway kinase-extracellular signal-regulated kinase (MEK) inhibitors; extracellular signal-regulated kinase is (ERK) inhibitors.[2]

SIROLIMUS (RAPAMYCIN)

The literature on Sirolimus and its efficacy is equivocal.

They reported a reduction in cellulitis and incidence of hospitalizations with cellulitis-related complications. The adverse effects of therapy were—metabolic toxicity (3%), gastro-intestinal

disturbance (3%), and blood/bone marrow abnormalities (27%). Not all the patients receiving therapy had a genetic test for the PIK3CA mutation confirmed. So, treatment was based on clinical considerations. Sirolimus' current indications for therapy are for pain, lesion enlargement, vesicular ulcerations, bone erosion and expansion, bleeding, airway compression, hematologic abnormalities, and complex symptomatic cases.[10–25,26,27]

Rapamycin

mTOR [10,11,24,25]

mTOR is a downstream enzyme in the PIK3CA pathway. Rapamycin is a chemotherapeutic agent derivative of streptomyces hygroscopicus bacteria, a macrolide used for targeted therapy to block the PIK3CA pathway. Rapamycin (Sirolimus) inhibits cellular proliferation.

Its use in head and neck vascular lesions has shown a qualitative reduction in size and side effects of bleeding and vesicular discharge.[28]

Gastrointestinal, general metabolic toxicity, blood dyscrasias, bone marrow suppression (even though one of the treatment indications is dyscrasias of hematological and marrow-derived cell function) were the reported adverse effects of the medications.

Other studies with–MEK1/2 (MAP2K1) GF. RTK.

Cellular membrane[29,30]

Anecdotal success with Sirolimus has been reported. Sirolimus' current indications for therapy are for pain, lesion enlargement, vesicular ulcerations, bone erosion and expansion, bleeding, airway compression, hematologic abnormalities, and complex symptomatic cases[2]

Genetic testing and advances in the understanding of pathogenesis have provided more direct and targeted therapeutics. However, the molecular abnormalities like cancer mutations and the phenotypic presentation disparity is intriguing. Nevertheless, mutations provide an objective molecular etiology to educate patients, families, and researchers with HNLM[3] knowledge for further work with a group of pathologies. Clinical pathways for standardized outcome measures and building data banks for systematic collection in medical trials is needed.[2]

Aggressive therapy needs more close followup and reporting. HNLM research makes precision-based treatment a possibility. Precision therapy-based treatment decision on specific molecular and genetic disorders is the future in vascular anamolies management. Biologic factors unique to an individual patient's rare conditions are always with meticulous risk-benefit ratio consideration.[3]

Table 3
"The mylohyoid artery branches proximal to the mandibular foramen. The anterior and middle superior alveolar arteries branch from the infraorbital artery proximal to the infraorbital foramen

Orbital and Extracranial Branches	Outer Diameter (mm)	Inner Diameter (mm)
Internal carotid artery (ICA)		
Ophthalmic artery[1]		1.35–1.37 ± 0.16–0.18
Orbital group		
Anterior ethmoidal artery[2]	0.88–0.92 ± 0.15–0.20	
Posterior ethmoidal artery[2]	0.63–0.66 ± 0.19–0.21	
Dorsal nasal artery[3,4]	0.74–0.88 ± 0.12–0.26	
Supratrochiear artery[3,4]	0.74–0.91 ± 0.17–0.20	
Supraorbital artery[4]	0.84 ± 0.16	
Superior and inferior medial palpebral arteries[4]	0.43 ± 0.13	
Lacrimal artery[5]	1.02–1.03 ± 0.16–0.17	
Superior and inferior lateral palpebral arteries, zygomati- cofacial artery, zygomaticotemporal artery[6,7]		
Ocular group		
Ciliary arteries		
Central retinal artery		
Muscular branches		
Arteries and Branches	Outer Diameter (mm)	Inner Diameter (mm)
External carotid artery (ECA)		
Superior thyroid artery[8–11]	2.1–3.53 ± 1.17–1.4	1.4–1.9 ± 0.3–0.7
Infrahyoid branch, superior laryngeal branch, sternomastoid branch, cricothyroid branch, glandular branches[12]		
Ascending pharyngeal artery[13,14]	1.4–1.54 ± 0.25–0.3	
Posterior meningeal artery, pharyngeal branches, inferior tympanic artery		
Lingual artery[8–11]	2.2–3.06 ± 0.65–1.L	1.6–1.8 ± 0.4
Deep lingual artery, sublingual artery, dorsal lingual branches, suprahyoid branch		
Facial artery[8–11]	2.7–3.35 ± 0.68–1.6	1.9–2.2 ± 0.4–0.5
Cervical branches: ascending palatine artery, tonsillar branch, submental artery, glandular branchesFacial branches: inferior labial, superior labial, inferior alar artery, lateral nasal artery, angular artery, forehead branch[15,16]		
External carotid artery (ECA)		
Occipital artery[17,18]	1.9–2.6	
SCM branches, meningeal branch, occipital branches, auricular branch, descending branch[19]		
Posterior auricular artery[20,21]	0.7–1.2	
StyJomastoid artery, stapedial artery, auricular branch, occipital branch, parotid branch		
Maxillary artery[10,22–24]	3.2–3.67 ± 0.07	2.1–2.3 ± 0.3–0.7

See table

		Outer Diameter (mm)	Inner Diameter (mm)
Superficial temporal artery[9,10,25]		2–2.73 ± 0.51–1.4	1.7 ± 0.4–0.5
Transverse facial artery, zygomatico-orbital artery, middle temporal artery, anterior auricular branch, frontal branches, parietal branch			

Divisions and Branches	Foramina	Outer Diameter (mm)	Inner Diameter (mm)
Maxillary artery			
Mandibular segment[23,24]		3.67 ± 0.07	2.1 ± 0.7
Deep auricular artery[23]	Squamotympanic fissure	1.0 ± 0.09	
Anterior tympanic artery[23]	Petrotympanic fissure	0.7 ± 0.002	
Middle meningeal artery[23,24]	Foramen spinosum	2.53 ± 0.38	1.2 ± 0.2
Accessory meningeal artery[23]	Foramen ovale	1.9 ± 0.22	
Inferior alveolar artery[23,24]	Mandibular foramen	1.3 ± 0.07	0.6 ± 0.1
Mylohyoid artery"			
Mental artery	Mental foramen		
Pterygoid segment[23]		3.24 ± 0.2	
Anterior deep temporal artery[23,24]		1.45 ± 0.10	0.7 ± 0.2
Posterior deep temporal artery[23,24]		1.48 ± 0.01	0.7 ± 0.1
Masseteric artery[23]		1.03 ± 0.02	
Buccal artery[23,24]		1.05 ± 0.07	0.6 ± 0.2
Pterygoid branches[23]		0.7 ± 0.003	
Pterygopalatine segment[23]		2.75 ± 0.04	
Descending palatine artery	Greater palatine canal		
Greater palatine artery[23]	Greater palatine foramen	0.71	
Les er palatine artery	Le ser palatine foramina		
Posterior superior alveolar artery[23,24]	Pterygomaxillary fissure	1.31 ± 0.07	1.0 ± 0.2
Infraorbital artery[23,24]	Infraorbital foramen	1.3 ± 0.08	1.0 ± 0.3
Anterior and middle superior alveolar arteriesb			
Sphenopalatine artery[23,24]	Sphenopalatine foramen	1.76 ± 0.48	1.2 ± 0.2
Lateral posterior nasal branches			
Posterior septa! branches			
Pharyngeal artery	Pharyngeal (palatovaginal) canal		
Artery of the pterygoid canal (Vidian artery)[23]	Pterygoid canal	0.7 ± 0.005	

Adopted from: Nair, Chandra Management of Head and Neck Vascular Lesions: A Guide for Surgeons, Springer Nature, Edition 1, May 2022; https://doi.org/10.1007/978-981-15-2321-2; ISBN978-981-15-2320-5.

In lesions where the RAS/RAF/MAPK/ERK pathway plays a significant role (eg, CM, CMAVM1 and 2, PG, NICH, RICH, and verrucous venous malformation), other inhibitors are considered. There are conceivable tests of BRAF (vemurafenib) or MEK inhibitor (trametinib), which are used to treat metastatic BRAF-mutated melanoma.[10,11] Because many kinase inhibitors have variable affinities to several intracellular proteins, and multiple cross-talks occur between signaling pathways, numerous studies are needed to characterize the most efficient modalities. In HHT, receptor mutations lead to decreased BMP signaling, and this may lead in turn to an increase in angiogenic response. Thus,

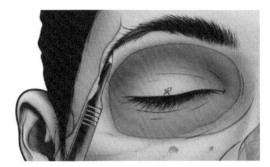

Fig. 5. Supraorbital approach with incisions in the hairline. (All right reserved to Brishank Pratop © 2021.)

these patients could benefit from antiangiogenic agents, such as bevacizumab. However, diminished ALK activity also leads to increased PTEN phosphorylation and inactivation. There is subse-quent PI3K/AKT activation. Rapamycin and other PI3K/AKT inhibitors may thus prove to be efficacious.[23]

Other general angiogenesis inhibitors, such as thalidomide or bevacizumab, the anti-VEGF antibody, may also be useful.[2] They can inhibit VEGF action, whatever the underlying cause for expression may be. For example, they reduce nosebleeds in patients with HHT. The pathophysiology of GVMs is a little unclear. If earlier data hold, the TGF-ß pathway might serve as a target, in addition to modulation of mTOR.[1,5,24,31–33]

GENERAL, SURGICAL, AND FUNCTIONAL ANATOMY FOR VASCULAR LESIONS OF HEAD AND NECK

Vessel and luminal dimensions (**Fig. 4** and **Table 3**)

The surgical approaches mentioned later are according to the Sanjiv Nair and colleagues' classification[2] (**Box 5**).

SUPRA ORBITAL APPROACH

A commonly used approach in the upper face is the supraorbital approach, which provides access to the frontozygomatic area. The incision is placed within the eyebrow hair (**Fig. 5**) and made through the skin and subcutaneous tissue till periosteum.

Periosteum integrity should be maintained so as to avoid herniation of the lacrimal gland. This approach is commonly used for the type 2 subcutaneous/juxta muscular lesions.[2]

UPPER EYELID APPROACH

Another approach that gained popularity due to its esthetic outcome is the upper eyelid approach also known as the supra-tarsal fold approach. This approach provides access to the upper bony orbit and can be used to excise tumors of soft tissue around the upper eye. This approach can be used for the type 1 Muscular/cutaneous, type 2 subcutaneous/juxta muscular lesions.[33]

VISOR INCISION

Submandibular, submental, and cervical parts of the head and neck are accessible through the cervical visor incision (**Fig. 6**). The flap is raised in a sub-platysmal plane all the way to the lower border of the mandible. This is suitable for type 3 glandular lesions.

Vascular lesions present in the subcutaneous plane (type II), Submandibular Gland (type III), deep to mylohyoid, and sternocleidomastoid (SCM), and supraclavicular region can be accessed. The posterior retraction of the SCM exposes the contents of the carotid sheath (common carotid artery, internal jugular vein, and vagus nerve). Control

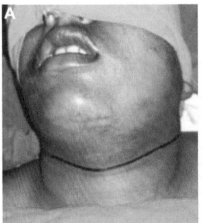
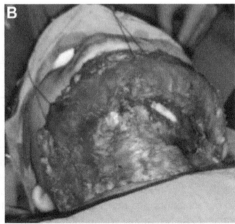

Fig. 6. The visor incision is an ample access to the neck, mandible, skull base and parotid areas. (*A*) skin incision (*B*) elevation of the skin and platysma flap elevation to the inferior border of the mandible.

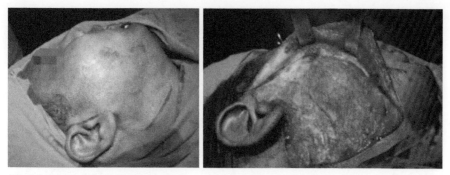

Fig. 7. Modified facelift incision (SMAS layer) for parotid and lesions of pre-auricular region.

of external carotid can be achieved as well through this approach.[34–36]

SUBMANDIBULAR APPROACH

These approaches are for lesions usually deep to the superficial musculoaponeurotic system layer but superficial to the mylohyoid and facial muscles and cannot be accessed intra-orally (refer to **Fig. 7**). The layers encountered in this region are skin, subcutaneous tissue, platysma muscle which extends from subcutaneous tissue of periclavicular region to insert into symphysis menti and merge with orbicularis oris. The capsule of the submandibular gland and the submandibular node can also be encountered here.

This is suitable for type 3 glandular lesions.[37]

MANDIBULAR ACCESS OSTEOTOMY[15]

The incision is placed in the submandibular skin crease as described previously and extended anteriorly in a wavy curve toward the mid-part of the chin, follows the submental skin crease laterally and continuing around the bulbous part of the chin onto the lower part of the face (**Fig. 8**A–E).

The mandibulotomy allows access to lesions in the deep lobe of parotid, parapharynx, and infratemporal fossa suitable for type IV and type V lesions.

WEBBER-FERGUSSON APPROACH

The Webber-Fergusson's incision and its modifications are used for approach to the anterior

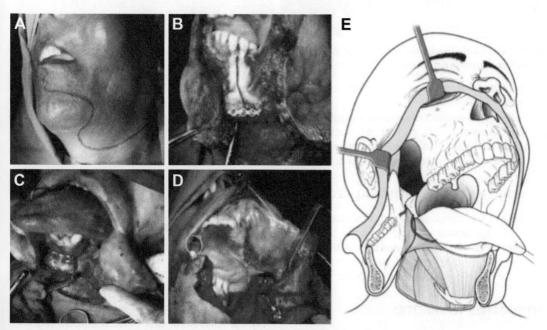

Fig. 8. Mandibular access osteotomy. (*A*) Skin marking of the incision (*B*) Mini-plate adapted prior to osteotomy (*B*) Mandible swung laterally after stripping muscles (*E*) Diagrammatic illustration of the procedure. (All right reserved to Brishank Pratop © 2021.)

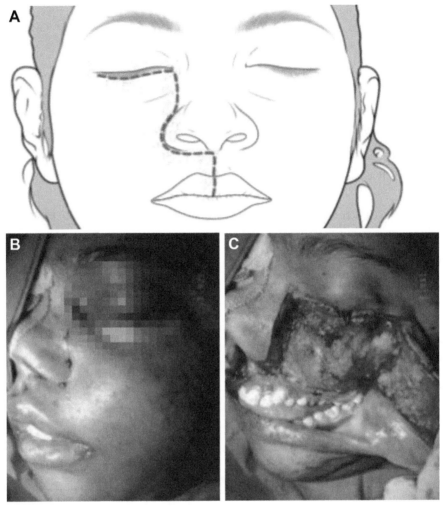

Fig. 9. (*A-C*) Dieffenbach's modification of Weber-Fergusson's approach. (*A*) Incision outline (*B,C*) Intraoperative incision and exposure. (All right reserved to Brishank Pratop © 2021.)

maxilla[24]; another approach is the midface degloving incision.[25] Ref **Fig. 9**.

The Weber–Fergusson incision is suitable for superficial lesions which cannot be approached intraorally or when wide excision of the maxilla is required for type IV intraosseous lesions.[15]

APPROACHES TO THE TEMPORAL REGION

Laterally in the temporal region, vascular lesions over the temporalis muscle warrant a lateral approach.(**Fig. 10**). This provides access to temporal region, malar area, and the temporomandibular region for which it was primarily designed.[2]

APPROACHES TO PAROTID

Approach to the temporomandibular joint (TMJ) is done through a Blair[13] incision (later modified by Bailey).[14] The superficial lobe of the parotid gland,

enclosed in the parotid masseteric fascia, overlaps the capsule of the TMJ in front of the external auditory meatus, hence the modified incision is used to access the intraglandular lesions (type III).[32]

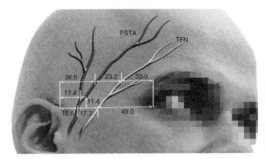

Fig. 10. Relations of facial nerve in temporal region (in mm). *Adapted from* Nair & Chandra, Management of Head and Neck Vascular Lesions-A Guide for Surgeons.2022.

CLINICS CARE POINTS

- Vascular anomalies have a "dynamic life-cycle". Biological syndrome-based grouping was logistical convenience, but with mutational foundations, the syndromes are reclassified.

- Between vascular tumors and malformations, tumors are more common, but you may encounter 'malformation' more often as they persist and need varied care. Patients usually present with multiple earlier investigations and interventions.

- Vascular anomalies—'group' of different entities of varied etio-pathological which may not share same treatments approaches.

- Airway/vision must be a consideration in managing head and neck anomalies, especially with syndromes and segmental presentations.

- Great potential for molecular and genetic research in this field-so multispecialty clinics save tissue samples for research laboratories for discovering targeted therapies.

REFERENCES

1. Mulliken JB, Glowacki J. Hemangiomas and vascular malformations in infants and children: a classification based on endothelial characteristics. P Reconstr Surg 1982;69(3):412–22.
2. Sanjiv C. Nair Srinivasa R. Chandra. Management of Head and Neck Vascular Lesions-A Guide for Surgeons.2022.
3. Waner M, Suen JY. Hemangiomas and vascular malformations of the head and neck. New York: Wiley-Liss; 1999.
4. Nair SC. Vascular anomalies of the head and neck region. J Maxillofac Oral Surg 2018;17:1–12.
5. Ethunandan M, Mellor TK. Hemangiomas and vascu- lar malformations of the maxillofacial region – review. Br J Maxillofac Surg 2006;44:263–72.
6. Bischoff J. Progenitor cells in infantile hemangioma. J Craniofac Surg 2009;20(Suppl 1):695.
7. Enjolras O, Mulliken JB. The current management of vascular birthmarks. Pediatr Dermatol 1993;10:311.
8. Martinez-Perez D, Fein NA, Boon LM, et al. Not all hemangiomas look like strawberries: uncommon presentations of the most common tumor of infancy. Pediatr Dermatol 1995;12:1–6.
9. Nair SC, Spencer NJ, Nayak KP, et al. Surgical management of vascular lesions of the head and neck: a review of 115 cases. Int J Oral Maxillofac Surg 2011; 40(6):577–83.
10. Padia R, Zenner K, Bly R, et al. Clinical application of molecular genetics in lymphatic malformations. Laryngoscope Investig Otolaryngol 2019;4(1): 170–3.
11. Greene AK, Goss JA. Vascular anomalies: from a clin- icohistologic to a genetic framework. Plast Reconstr Surg 2018;141:709e–17e.
12. Kinross KM, Montgomery KG, Kleinschmidt M, et al. An activating PIK3CA mutation coupled with Pten loss is sufficient to initiate ovarian tumorigenesis in mice. J Clin Invest 2012;122:553–7.
13. Samuels Y, Wang Z, Bardelli A, et al. High frequency of mutations of the PIK3CA gene in human cancers. Science 2004;304:554.
14. Samuels Y, Ericson K. Oncogenic PI3K and its role in cancer. Curr Opin Oncol 2006;18:77–82.
15. Luks VL, Kamitaki N, Vivero MP. Lymphatic and other vascular malformative/overgrowth disorders are caused by somatic mutations in PIK3CA. J Pediatr.
16. 2015;166(1048–1054):e1041–5.
17. Keppler-Noreuil KM, Rios JJ, Parker VE, et al. PIK3CA- related overgrowth spectrum (PROS): diagnos- tic and testing eligibility criteria, differential diagnosis, and evaluation. Am J Med Genet 2015; 167A:287–95.
18. Vignot S, Faivre S, Aguirre D, et al. mTOR- targeted therapy of cancer with rapamycin derivatives. Ann Oncol 2005;16:525–37.
19. Sasongko TH, Ismail NF, Zabidi-Hussin Z. Rapamycin and rapalogs for tuberous sclerosis complex. Cochrane Database Syst Rev 2016;7:CD011272.
20. Alemi AS, Rosbe KW, Chan DK, et al. Airway response to sirolimus therapy for the treatment of complex pediatric lymphatic malformations. Int J Pediatr Otorhinolaryngol 2015;79:2466–9.
21. Lagreze WA, Joachimsen L, Gross N, et al. Sirolimus-induced regression of a large orbital lymphangioma. Orbit 2018;38:1–2.
22. Yesil S, Tanyildiz HG, Bozkurt C, et al. Single-center experience with sirolimus therapy for vascular malformations. Pediatr Hematol Oncol 2016;33:219–25.
23. Yesil S, Bozkurt C, Tanyildiz HG, et al. Successful treatment of macroglossia due to lymphatic malformation with sirolimus. Ann Otol Rhinol Laryngol 2015;124:820–3.
24. Venot Q, Blanc T, Rabia SH, et al. Targeted therapy in patients with PIK3CA-related overgrowth syndrome. Nature 2018;558:540–6.
25. Cramer SL, Wei S, Merrow AC, et al. Gorham- Stout disease success- fully treated with Sirolimus and zoledronic acid therapy. J Pediatr Hematol Oncol 2016;38:e129–32.
26. Dvorakova V, Rea D, O'Regan GM, et al. Generalized lymphatic anomaly successfully treated with long-term, low-dose Sirolimus. Pediatr Dermatol 2018;35(4):533–4.

27. Mulliken JB, Fishman SJ, Burrows PE. Vascular anomalies. Curr Probl Surg 2000;37:517.

28. Saint-Jean M, Léauté-Labrèze C, Mazereeuw-Hautier J, et al. Propranolol for treatment of ulcerated infantile hemangiomas. J Am Acad Dermatol 2011;64:827.

29. Nair SC, Chandra SR. Management of head and neck vascular lesions: a Guide for Surgeons. Edition 1. Springer Nature; 2022. https://doi.org/10.1007/978-981-15-2321-2. ISBN978-981-15-2320-5.

30. Nair SC. Vascular Anomalies of the Head and Neck Region. J Maxillofac Oral Surg 2018;17:1–12.

31. Chandra SR, Nair S. History, terminology, and classifications of vascular anomalies-pages 1-9, management of head and neck vascular lesions: a Guide for Surgeons. Edition 1. Springer Nature; 2022. https://doi.org/10.1007/978-981-15-2321-2. ISBN978-981-15-2320-5.

32. Chandra SR, Kumar B, Shroff S, et al. Pathogenesis, genetics, and molecular developments in vascular lesion therapy and diagnosis, pages 11-27; management of head and neck vascular lesions: a Guide for Surgeons. Edition 1. Springer Nature; 2022. https://doi.org/10.1007/978-981-15-2321-2. ISBN978-981-15-2320-5.

33. Chandra SR, Yu L, Ghodke B. Radiological diagnosis of head and neck vascular Anomalies,pages 49-65, management of head and neck vascular lesions: a Guide for Surgeons. Edition 1. Springer Nature; 2022. https://doi.org/10.1007/978-981-15-2321-2. ISBN978-981-15-2320-5.

34. Chandra SR, Kumar J, Nair SC. Medical management of vascular lesions: current and the future, pages 67-103, management of head and neck vascular lesions: a Guide for Surgeons. Edition 1. Springer Nature; 2022. https://doi.org/10.1007/978-981-15-2321-2. ISBN978-981-15-2320-5.

35. Chandra SR, Shroff S, Curry S, et al. General, surgical, and functional anatomy for vascular lesions of head and neck, pages 105-135; management of head and neck vascular lesions: a Guide for Surgeons. Edition 1. Springer Nature; 2022. https://doi.org/10.1007/978-981-15-2321-2. ISBN978-981-15-2320-5.

36. Nair SC, Shroff S, Chandra SR. Surgical management, pages 137-157, management of head and neck vascular lesions: a Guide for Surgeons. Edition 1. Springer Nature; 2022. https://doi.org/10.1007/978-981-15-2321-2. ISBN978-981-15-2320-5.

37. Burt J, Rodriguez-Vasquez J, Ghodke B, et al. The role of interventional radiology, pages 67-103; management of head and neck vascular lesions: a Guide for Surgeons. Edition 1. Springer Nature; 2022. https://doi.org/10.1007/978-981-15-2321-2. ISBN978-981-15-2320-5.

Dermatologic Review in Pediatric Vascular Lesions

Helena Vidaurri de la Cruz, MD[a,b,c],*, Felipe Velasquez Valderrama, MD[d], Rosalía Ballona Chambergo, MD[d]

KEYWORDS

- Skin examination • Vascular anomalies • Skin tumors • Developmental defects • Atypical infections
- Multidisciplinary management

KEY POINTS

- Vascular anomalies (VAs) frequently affect the skin.
- Accurate diagnosis of any skin lesion is key to successful management.
- Pediatric dermatologists are specially trained to distinguish VAs on the skin from their mimickers.
- VA clinics must include pediatric dermatologist to aid in the diagnosis, management, follow-up, and integral treatment of patients.

INTRODUCTION

Estimated prevalence of vascular anomaly (VA) is 4.5% of all pediatric dermatology consultations, 5% of all newborns may have a VA,[1] and up to 12% of Caucasian infants show a vascular skin lesion.[2] The latest classification produced by the International Society for the Study of Vascular Anomalies (ISSVA) in 2018[3] considers vascular tumors (VTs) and vascular malformations (VMs) as 2 different groups. ISSVA's classification is being currently revised. VTs are cellular proliferations that escape the tissue's signals for normal cell growth, cell differentiation, and death. However, VMs are developmental defects of the blood or lymphatic vessels due to somatic mutations in genes belonging to the phosphatidylinositol-3-kinase/Akt kinase/mammalian target of rapamycin (mTOR) (PI3K/AKT/mTOR) and Rat sarcoma/mitogen-activated protein kinases vasculogenesis signaling pathways, which may affect not only vascular tissue but also soft tissue or other organs, including bone.[4] VT clinical behavior depends on

their specific cell line, for example, infantile hemangiomas have a characteristic history of proliferation and involution; kaposiform hemangioendotheliomas keep growing and may produce Kasabach Merritt phenomenon; pyogenic granulomas grow very quickly and have spontaneous bleeding; and angiosarcomas have metastatic potential. VM progressively dilate, causing soft tissue hypertrophy, bleeding, coagulopathy, failure to thrive, or high-output cardiac failure.

Because VAs may present with different clinical features, patients with VAs should be cared for by several specialists, ideally constituting a VA clinic. Participants in such clinics must include pediatricians, pediatric dermatologists, hemato-oncologists, geneticists, pediatric surgeons, plastic surgeons, angiologists, interventional radiologists, and any other specialist that is needed, for example, gynecologist for VAs affecting the pelvis in female patients, ophthalmologist for those affecting the eyelids or the eye, and so forth.[5]

History and physical examination (H&PE) of the suspected VA are the main elements to arrive to

[a] Department of Pediatrics, Hospital General de México Dr. Eduardo Liceaga, O.D. Health Ministry, Mexico City, Mexico; [b] National Autonomous University of Mexico; [c] Society for Pediatric Dermatology, Latin American Society of Pediatric Dermatology, European Academy of Dermatology and Venereology, International Society of Pediatric Dermatology, Mexican Academy of Pediatrics, Mexican Academy of Dermatology; [d] Instituto Nacional de Salud del Niño de Breña, Lima, Peru
* Corresponding author. Pediatric Dermatology Clinic, Department of Pediatrics, Querétaro 147-406, Col. Roma, Cuauhtémoc CDMX 06700.
E-mail address: Helena.vidaurri@gmail.com

Oral Maxillofacial Surg Clin N Am 36 (2024) 49–60
https://doi.org/10.1016/j.coms.2023.09.008

the correct diagnosis in 90% of patients.[6] Imaging studies are useful to assess the influence on other organs, associated developmental field disorders, and to distinguish the lesion from other diseases.

Every patient with a suspected VA affecting the skin should be examined by a pediatric dermatologist or a dermatologist with interest and experience in the management of VA to achieve several goals.

1. Perform a complete H&PE including the evaluation of physical growth and development.
2. Consider differential diagnoses: benign and malignant tumors, cysts, and closure defects of embryonic structures, and treat accordingly.
3. Distinguish among different VAs: infantile hemangioma, congenital hemangiomas, other VTs (kaposiform hemangioendothelioma, tufted angioma, and even angiosarcoma), venous malformations, lymphatic malformations, and arterio-venous malformations, and treat accordingly.
4. Consider medical treatment options, such as propranolol for hemangiomas, rapamycin for lymphatic and venous malformations, thalidomide for arteriovenous malformations, alpelisib for phosphatidylinositol-4,5-bisphosphate 3-kinase catalytic subunit alpha (PIK3CA)-related overgrowth syndromes, or mitogen-activated protein kinase (MEK) inhibitors for specific lesions.[7]
5. Consider a skin biopsy in lesions with H&PE suggestive of diagnoses different than VA, in VA with insufficient response to treatments, and for tissue genomic tests.
6. Consider pulsed dye laser treatment in capillary malformations.
7. Referral to diagnostic radiology for sonography,[8,9] computed tomography scan, MRI, or angiography.[10]
8. Referral to pediatric surgery for other treatment options in VA: removal of redundant skin in involuted hemangiomas and excision in noninvoluting congenital hemangiomas or other vascular anomalies (VAs).[11]
9. Referral to interventional radiology for other treatment options in VA: embolization in noninvoluting congenital hemangiomas, sclerosis in venous malformations, or sclerosis/embolization in arteriovenous malformations.[12,13]
10. Referal to other specialties (genetics, pediatric ophthalmology, pediatric ofthopedics, pediatric neurology, pediatric hemato-oncology, etc) to perform a complete evaluation and treat associated syndromes of complications, such as PHACE or LUMBAR.PHACE: posterior fossa anomalies, hemangioma, arterial anomalies of the brain and aorta, cardiac,

eye and sternal anomalies). LUMBAR (lower body hemangioma or other skin defects, urogenital anomalies, ulceration, myelopathy, bone deformities, anorectal malformations, arterial and renal anomalies).[14]

DIFFERENTIAL DIAGNOSIS OF SUSPECTED VASCULAR ANOMALY

Many skin diseases present with red, blue, or purple plaques or nodules, just as VAs do. Moreover, skin-colored nodules may be due to VAs, especially lymphatic malformations, but may also be due to other skin diseases or tumors (**Tables 1–4**). To treat each of these lesions appropriately, several differential diagnoses must be considered.[15–34]

ILLUSTRATIVE CASES

1. A 12-year-old female patient with progressive soft tissue growth of the left cheek and left lower lip in the former 3 years. Angiography of both carotid arteries showed a slow flow arteriovenous malformation (AVM) on the left lower lip and left cheek. Embolization of the left lower lip artery and 5 venous scleroses were performed with 40% of volume reduction of the AVM. We prescribed thalidomide after a thorough discussion of potential benefits and adverse effects with the patient and her parents. After 4 months of treatment, the patient, and her mother notice less volume increase of the AVM with physical activity (**Fig. 1**).
2. A 1-month-old male patient with congenital VT on the occipital region. The patient required treatment of hypoglycemia and neonatal sepsis. He was referred to pediatric dermatology by 2 months of age; in the meantime, the lesion had decreased in size without any specific treatment. Ultrasonography of the lesion showed several tortuous vascular structures. He was diagnosed with a rapid involuting congenital hemangioma (RICH) and was followed monthly until complete resolution by 1 year of age (**Fig. 2**).
3. A 13-year-old female patient with a venous malformation on the anterior neck and sternal region. The VM was evident at 10 years of age. She was treated with sclerosing agents with good results; we then prescribed rapamycin and the VM decreased its size further. Multidisciplinary treatment has led to best results (**Fig. 3**).
4. A 3-month-old female patient with a left breast infantile hemangioma at proliferative stage. She has received 6 months of oral propranolol, and

Table 1
Mimickers of vascular anomalies: benign skin tumors and cysts

Benign Skin Tumors and cysts	Cell Origin	Localization	Clinical Features	Evolution	Age	Frequency	Treatment
Pilomatricoma[15]	Hair follicle matrix	Head, neck, trunk, and upper limbs	Asymptomatic, subcutaneous polyhedric, firm or hard, mobile tumor Skin colored, bluish, or reddish 0.5–6 cm in diameter	Slow growth, sometimes spontaneous involution	School-aged children and teenagers	Common	Surgical excision
Spitz nevus[16]	Melanocytes	Mainly head, neck, lower limbs but may occur elsewhere	Asymptomatic, skin-colored, red, pink, brown or black tumor	Rapid growth over some months, occasionally may bleed, or be painful	Children and young adults	Common in Caucasian children	Surgical excision
Neurothekeoma[17]	Peripheral nerve sheath	Head, neck, trunk, and upper limbs	Asymptomatic, reddish cutaneous tumor Myxoid, cellular, and mixed types Cellular type may have atypia	Rapid growth over some months	School-aged children, teenagers, adults	Uncommon	Surgical excision

(continued on next page)

Table 1
(*continued*)

Benign Skin Tumors and cysts	Cell Origin	Localization	Clinical Features	Evolution	Age	Frequency	Treatment
Epidermoid (inclusion) cyst[18]	Keratinocytes and epidermal entrapment	Any location	Asymptomatic skin-colored spherical cyst with a central punctum. Some may be associated with fusion defects of embryonic structures	Slow growth	Any age	Common	Surgical excision
Trichilemmal cyst[19]	Outer root sheath of the hair follicle	Scalp, limbs, and neck	Asymptomatic spherical, rubbery subcutaneous cysts of skin color, or pink	Slow growth	Teenagers and adults	5%–10% of the population	Surgical excision
Xanthogranuloma[20]	Non–Langerhans cell histiocytes	Head, neck, and limbs	Asymptomatic reddish-orange tumor 0.5–3 cm	Self-limited growth, spontaneous involution	First year of life	1.5% of pediatric tumors	Active surveillance or surgical excision
Eccrine poroma[21]	Intraepidermal portion of the eccrine sweat duct	Palms, soles, chest, eye, and buttocks	Painful red-colored or skin-colored tumor	Slow growth	Adults	rare	Surgical excision

Myofibroma[22]	Myofibroblast	Trunk and limbs	Elastic, hard, reddish to yellowish tumor	Congenital or slow growth, self-limited growth, spontaneous involution. When multiple lesions, systemic involvement may occur	First 2 years of life	common	Active surveillance, occasionally, systemic treatment
Fibrous hamartoma[23]	Fibroblastic/ myofibroblastic cells, mature adipose tissue, highly vascular, and myxoid nodules	Axillary region, upper arm, upper trunk, inguinal region, and external genital area	Asymptomatic, subcutaneous tumor	Congenital or slow growth	Congenital or first year of life	Rare	Surgical excision

Table 2
Mimickers of vascular anomalies: developmental defects

Developmental Defects	Cell Origin	Localization	Clinical Features	Evolution	Age	Frequency	Treatment
Dermoid cyst[24]	Epidermal entrapment along embryonic fusion lines	Head, neck, and trunk	Asymptomatic, spherical subcutaneous cyst of skin color	Congenital	Newborns, children, and teenagers	Rare: 3/10,000 pediatric patients	Surgical excision
Nasal glioma[25]	Cerebral heterotopia	Nasal dorsum	Compressible smooth mass	Congenital	Newborns	Rare	Surgical excision
Meningocele[26]	Failure of neurulation	Posterior midline and facial midline	Subcutaneous masses with loss of neurologic function distal to the lesion level	Congenital	Newborns	1:1000 pregnancies	Multidisciplinary
Preauricular cysts[27]	Failure of fusion of branchial arches	Cheek	Asymptomatic spherical subcutaneous cyst of skin color	Congenital	Newborns, children, and teenagers	0.02%–5% of general population	Surgical excision
Thyroglossal duct cysts[28]	Thyroid remnants	Anterior neck, base of the tongue, and suprasternal	Painless swelling that moves when patient swallows	Congenital	Mainly younger than 10-year-olds	7% of general population	Surgical excision
Bronchogenic cyst[29]	Bronchial epithelium	Neck	Slow growing symptomatic or asymptomatic tumor, depending on the proximity to the airway	Congenital	Newborns, children, occasionally teenagers and adults	Rare	Surgical excision

Table 3
Mimickers of vascular anomalies: malignant skin tumors

Malignant Tumors	Cell Origin	Localization	Clinical Features	Evolution	Age	Frequency	Treatment
Amelanotic melanoma[30]	Melanocytes	Any location	Red-colored or skin-colored tumor of recent appearance and active growth, sometimes with easy bleeding, and any diameter	Recent appearance and active growth	Any age	All melanomas: All phototypes, mainly in I–II; 1%–3% of pediatric malignancies; Amelanotic melanoma is more frequent in children aged younger than 10 years	Surgical excision and oncology management
Dermatofibrosarcoma protuberans[31]	Fibroblasts	Trunk, proximal extremities, and rarely in head and neck	Nodular: Pink, reddish, flesh or bluish color firm tumor	Slow growth	Any age	Rare	Surgical excision and oncology management
Rhabdomyosarcoma[32]	Skeletal muscle tissue	Head, neck, limbs, and trunk	One or multiple lesions Alveolar or embryonal: erythematous firm tumor	Rapid growth	Any age	Primary cutaneous: rare Nonprimary cutaneous: more frequent	Surgical excision and oncology management
Infantile fibrosarcoma[32]	Fibroblasts	Any location, mainly lower extremities	Asymptomatic skin colored or with hemorrhagic foci	Rapid growth	First year of life, 30% congenital	Most frequent malignant soft tissue tumor of skin and adipose tissue in children aged younger than 1 year	Surgical excision and oncology management
Other soft tissue sarcomas[32]	Mesenchymal tissue	Any location	Asymptomatic skin-colored or reddish tumors	Rapid growth	Any age	Rare	Surgical excision and oncology management
Leukemia cutis[33]	White blood cells	Any location	Red, brown, or purple nodules	Rapid growth	Any age	Rare	Biopsy and hemato-oncology management

Table 4
Mimickers of vascular anomalies: infectious diseases

Skin Infections	Causal Agent	Localization	Clinical Features	Evolution	Age	Frequency	Treatment
Bacillary angiomatosis[34]	*Bartonella quintana* or *Bartonella henselae*	Face and extremities	Solitary or multiple, red-colored or flesh-colored papules, nodules, or tumors that are friable and easily bleeding. Can be accompanied by systemic disease	Initial phase: fever, hemolytic anemia, transient immunodeficiency Chronic phase: angiomatous lesions of long duration, with or without systemic symptoms	Any, vector transmitted	Neglected, reemergent disease, more frequent in populations in contact with arthropods and domestic animals	Biopsy and antibiotic treatment
Mycobacteriosis[35]	*Mycobacterium tuberculosis* and atypical mycobacteria	Neck, axilla and groin	Reddish, tender or nontender nodules	Slow growth	Any	Rare More common in immune-compromised or undernourished patients	Biopsy, antibiotic treatment

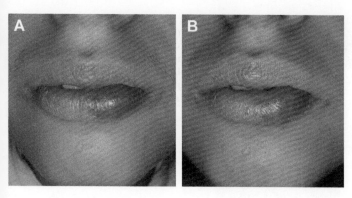

Fig. 1. 12-year-old female patient. (*A*) AVM after 1 embolization and 5 scleroses, before thalidomide. (*B*) AVM 4 months after thalidomide, notice less volume on lower left lip. (*Courtesy of* Dr Helena Vidaurri de la Cruz, MD.)

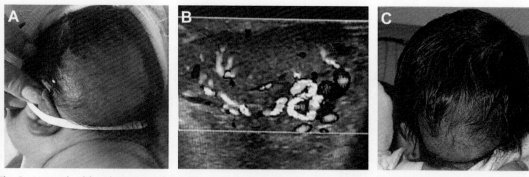

Fig. 2. 1-month-old male patient. (*A*) RICH on the occipital region. (*B*) Ultrasonography showing several tortuous vascular structures. (*C*) Same patient at 1 year of age. Management: active surveillance, no medication. Notice involution of RICH. (*Courtesy of* Dr Helena Vidaurri de la Cruz, MD.)

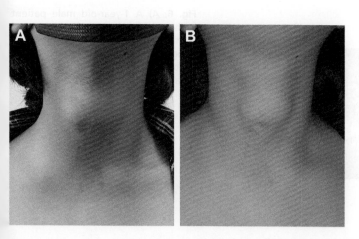

Fig. 3. 13-year-old female patient. (*A*) Venous malformation after 5 scleroses, before rapamycin. (*B*) Venous malformation after 2 additional scleroses and rapamycin for 7 months, notice volume decrease in the venous malformation. (*Courtesy of* Dr Helena Vidaurri de la Cruz, MD.)

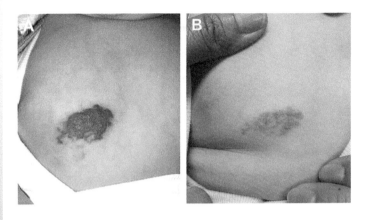

Fig. 4. Female patient with left breast hemangioma. (*A*) At 3 months of age, before oral propranolol. (*B*) At 9 months of age, after 6 months of oral propranolol, notice involution of infantile hemangioma. (*Courtesy of* Dr Helena Vidaurri de la Cruz, MD.)

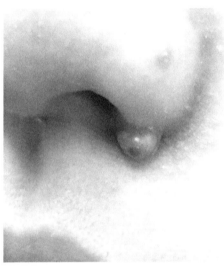

Fig. 5. 10-year-old female patient with red nodule beneath left nostril. Histopathology revealed a nodular neurothekeoma. (*Courtesy of* Dr Helena Vidaurri de la Cruz, MD.)

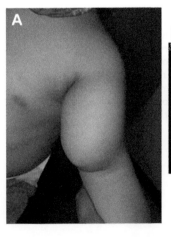

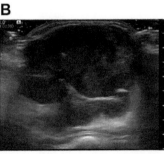

Fig. 6. *A*) A 1-year-old male patient with soft tissue progressive growth on the left arm since the first month of age. (*B*) Biopsy revealed an infantile fibrosarcoma. (*Courtesy of* Dr Helena Vidaurri de la Cruz, MD.)

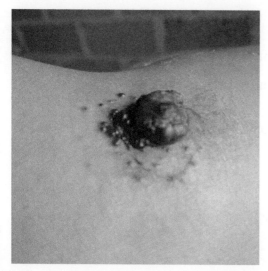

Fig. 7. 13-year-old female patient with agminated red nodules on the right supraclavicular region, with progressive growth in the former 6 months. Histopathology revealed pyogenic granuloma. (*Courtesy of* Dr Helena Vidaurri de la Cruz, MD.)

the hemangioma has involuted progressively with excellent results (**Fig. 4**).

5. A 10-year-old female patient with a red nodule beneath her left nostril. The lesion had progressively grown in the former 3 months. Differential diagnoses included pyogenic granuloma, Spitz nevus, neurothekeoma, and pilomatrixoma. The lesion was completely excised. Histopathology revealed a nodular neurothekeoma (**Fig. 5**).

6. A 1-year-old male patient with soft tissue growth on the left arm since the first month of age. Due to low vascular flow evident on ultrasonography, the lesion was diagnosed as a hemangioma and the patient received propranolol at another institution without any response, and further growth of the lesion. Differential diagnoses included vascular anomaly, soft tissue sarcoma, or soft tissue benign tumor. Biopsy revealed an infantile fibrosarcoma. Treatment included surgery, chemotherapy, and radiotherapy with excellent outcome (**Fig. 6**).

7. A 13-year-old female patient with agminated red nodules on her right supraclavicular region, which had progressively appeared and grown in the former 6 months without any systemic symptoms. Differential diagnoses included pyogenic granuloma, soft tissue sarcoma, and amelanotic melanoma. Biopsy revealed pyogenic granuloma. The lesion was completely excised, and histopathology confirmed pyogenic granuloma (**Fig. 7**).

SUMMARY

VAs frequently affect the skin. Thorough skin exploration is key to arrive to a correct diagnosis of any suspected skin lesion, including VAs. Differential diagnosis of VAs includes benign and malignant tumors of the skin, soft tissue, and skin metastases, as well as developmental defects, and even atypical infections. Pediatric dermatologists are specially trained to distinguish among such diverse diseases, to treat most of them with topical and systemic medication, and to refer patients in need of surgical treatment or interventional radiology management.

CLINICS CARE POINTS

- When evaluating a bump on the skin, consider differentials: skin tumor, skin inflammatory and infectious diseases, VTs, VA, embryologic closure defects, and skin metastasis. If diagnosis is unclear, ask for a pediatric dermatology/dermatology consultation.

- When diagnosing VTs or VMs, consider multidisciplinary treatment, including medical, interventional, and surgical, to best serve the patient's interests.

- When caring for patients with VAs, consider their dynamic behavior. Even when VAs may seem controlled at any developmental stage of children, teenagers, and adults, they may change in the future, and they must be followed and treated accordingly.

DECLARATION OF INTERESTS

All authors state they have no financial or other interests related to the submitted publication.

DISCLOSURE

Authors do not have any financial or nonfinancial conflict of interrest to disclose.

ACKNOWLEDGMENT

We thank the patients and medical colleagues from the vascular anomaly clinics in our hospitals for all the knowledge they have shared with us while attending to these very complex phenotypes.

REFERENCES

1. Yilmaz L, Kacenelenbogen N. Les anomalies vasculaires cutanées chez l'enfant [Cutaneous vascular

anomalies in children]. Rev Med Brux 2015;36(4): 348–57.

2. MacFie CC, Jeffery SLA. Diagnosis of Vascular Skin Lesions in Children: An Audit and Review. Pediatr Dermatol 2008;25:7–12.

3. ISSVA Classification of Vascular Anomalies ©2018 International Society for the Study of Vascular Anomalies Available at "issva.org/classification" Accessed June 3, 2023.

4. Borst AJ, Hammill AM, Crary SE, et al. Barriers to Genetic Testing in Vascular Malformations. JAMA Netw Open 2023;6(5):e2314829.

5. Mathes EFD, Haggstrom AN, Dowd C, et al. Clinical Characteristics and Management of Vascular Anomalies: Findings of a Multidisciplinary Vascular Anomalies Clinic. Arch Dermatol 2004;140(8):979–83.

6. Theiler M, Wälchli R, Weibel L. Vascular anomalies – a practical approach. JDDG J der Deutschen Dermatol Gesellschaft 2013;11:397–405.

7. Dekeuleneer V, Seront E, Van Damme A, et al. Theranostic Advances in Vascular Malformations. J Invest Dermatol 2020;140(4):756–63.

8. Rodríguez Bandera AI, Sebaratnam DF, Feito Rodríguez M, et al. Cutaneous ultrasound and its utility in pediatric dermatology. Part I: Lumps, bumps, and inflammatory conditions. Pediatr Dermatol 2020;37: 29–39.

9. Rodríguez Bandera AI, Sebaratnam DF, Feito Rodríguez M, et al. Cutaneous ultrasound and its utility in *Pediatric Dermatology*: Part II—Developmental anomalies and vascular lesions. Pediatr Dermatol 2020;37:40–51.

10. Mamlouk MD, Danial C, McCullough WP. Vascular anomaly imaging mimics and differential diagnoses. Pediatr Radiol 2019;49(8):1088–103.

11. Goldenberg DC, Zatz RF. Surgical Treatment of Vascular Anomalies. Dermatol Clin 2022;40(4): 473–80.

12. Scollan ME, Azimov N, Garzon MC, et al. An overview of interventional radiology techniques for the diagnosis and management of vascular anomalies: Part 1. Pediatr Dermatol 2023;40(2):242–9.

13. Scollan ME, Azimov N, Garzon MC, et al. An overview of interventional radiology techniques for the diagnosis and management of vascular anomalies: Part 2. Pediatr Dermatol 2022;1–8. https://doi.org/10.1111/pde.15224.

14. Stefanko NS, Davies OMT, Beato MJ, et al. Hamartomas and midline anomalies in association with infantile hemangiomas, PHACE, and LUMBAR syndromes. Pediatr Dermatol 2020;37:78–85.

15. Jones CD, Ho W, Robertson BF, et al. Pilomatrixoma: A Comprehensive Review of the Literature. Am J Dermatopathol 2018;40(9):631–41.

16. Brown A, Sawyer JD, Neumeister MW. Spitz Nevus: Review and Update. Clin Plast Surg 2021;48(4): 677–86.

17. Massimo JA, Gasibe M, Massimo I, et al. Neurothekeoma: Report of two cases in children and review of the literature. Pediatr Dermatol 2020;37(1):187–9.

18. Hoang VT, Trinh CT, Nguyen CH, et al. Overview of epidermoid cyst. Eur J Radiol Open 2019;6:291–301.

19. He P, Cui LG, Wang JR, et al. Trichilemmal Cyst: Clinical and Sonographic Features. J Ultrasound Med 2019;38(1):91–6.

20. Hernández-San Martín MJ, Vargas-Mora P, Aranibar LJ. Xanthogranuloma: An Entity With a Wide Clinical Spectrum. Actas Dermosifiliogr (Engl Ed) 2020;111(9):725–33. English, Spanish.

21. Wankhade V, Singh R, Sadhwani V, et al. Eccrine poroma. Indian Dermatol Online J 2015;6(4):304–5.

22. Ogita A, Ansai SI. Infantile Myofibroma: Case Report and Review of the Literature. J Nippon Med Sch 2021;87(6):355–8.

23. Al-Ibraheemi A, Martinez A, Weiss SW, et al. Fibrous hamartoma of infancy: a clinicopathologic study of 145 cases, including 2 with sarcomatous features. Mod Pathol 2017;30(4):474–85.

24. Orozco-Covarrubias L, Lara-Carpio R, Saez-De-Ocariz M, et al. Dermoid cysts: a report of 75 pediatric patients. Pediatr Dermatol 2013;30(6):706–11.

25. Van Wyhe RD, Chamata ES, Hollier LH. Midline Craniofacial Masses in Children. Semin Plast Surg 2016;30(4):176–80.

26. Copp AJ, Greene ND. Neural tube defects–disorders of neurulation and related embryonic processes. Wiley Interdiscip Rev Dev Biol 2013 Mar-Apr;2(2):213–27.

27. Hills SE, Maddalozzo J. Congenital lesions of epithelial origin. Otolaryngol Clin North Am 2015;48(1): 209–23.

28. Taha A, Enodien B, Frey DM, et al. Thyroglossal Duct Cyst, a Case Report and Literature Review. Diseases 2022;10(1):7.

29. Nolasco-de la Rosa AL, Nuñez-Trenado LA, Román-Guzmán E, et al. Quiste broncogénico en cuello. Reporte de un caso y revisión de la bibliografía [Neck bronchogenic cyst. Case report and review of the literature]. Cir Cir 2016 May-Jun;84(3):235–9. Spanish.

30. Stefanaki C, Chardalias L, Soura E, et al. Paediatric melanoma. J Eur Acad Dermatol Venereol 2017; 31(10):1604–15.

31. Sleiwah A, Wright TC, Chapman T, et al. Dermatofibrosarcoma Protuberans in Children. Curr Treat Options Oncol 2022;23(6):843–54.

32. Drabent P, Fraitag S. Malignant Superficial Mesenchymal Tumors in Children. Cancers 2022;14(9): 2160.

33. Paquette GM, Cotter C, Huang JT. Pearls and updates: cutaneous signs of systemic malignancy. Curr Opin Pediatr 2022;34(4):367–73.

34. Lins KA, Drummond MR, Velho PE. Cutaneous manifestations of bartonellosis. An Bras Dermatol 2019; 94(5):594–602.

Management of Midfacial and Skull Vault Osseous Vascular Lesions

Madan Ethunandan, MDS, FRCS (OMFS), FDSRCS, FFDRCSI[a,b,]*

KEYWORDS

- Intraosseous vascular malformations • Venous malformations • Arteriovenous malformations
- Embolization • Virtual surgical planning

KEY POINTS

- Specific imaging features can help characterize the individual vascular lesions.
- Multidisciplinary management will enable best outcomes for this patient group.
- Virtual surgical planning, with surgical guides and patient-specific implants, is helpful in obtaining consistently excellent results.
- Eventual form and function (eg, binocular vision and dental rehabilitation) will have to be taken into account in managing periorbital and midface lesions.
- Embolization has a crucial role to play in the management of high-flow arteriovenous malformations.

Vascular anomalies have been historically poorly understood and the terminology used to describe them confusing and ambiguous. The descriptive terminology used in the past (port-wine stain, strawberry hemangioma, salmon patch) conjure up visual approximations to the lesions but have no correlation with the biological behavior or natural history of the lesions.[1] Since the seminal work of Mulliken and Glowacki, vascular lesions have been principally categorized as hemangiomas and vascular malformations.[2] Flow characteristics have further helped in categorizing the vascular lesions into high-flow and low-flow lesions.[3] The International Society for the Study of Vascular Anomalies (ISSVA) published a unified classification system for vascular anomalies in 1996, which were updated in 2007 and 2014, with the most recent update in 2018.[4] This classification system divides these lesions into vascular tumors and malformations. This classification is meant to represent the "state of art" in vascular anomalies classification, acknowledging that it will require modifications as new scientific information becomes available. The ISSVA classification does not include a separate category for intraosseous lesions, but Nair and colleagues classified vascular lesions according to their location and depth and included a separate category for intraosseous lesions.[5]

Although a widely accepted classification system for vascular lesions has existed for more than 30 years, there still continues to be widespread misuse of nomenclature and terminologies in the literature.[6,7] Hassanein and colleagues[7] evaluated the literature with the search word "haemangioma" and found that 71% (228 of 320) had misused this terminology; of the patients who were mislabeled, 21% received improper management. All the patients who were accurately diagnosed received appropriate management. It is vitally important that precise terminology is used to enable appropriate treatment.

[a] Oral & Maxillofacial Surgery, University Hospital Southampton, Tremona Road, Southampton, SO16 6YD, UK;
[b] Oral & Maxillofacial Surgery, Sri Ramchandra Institute of Higher Education and Research, Prour, Chennai, 600116, India
* Corresponsing author. Oral & Maxillofacial Surgery, University Hospital Southampton, Tremona Road, Southampton, SO16 6YD.
E-mail address: mgethu@hotmail.com

Oral Maxillofacial Surg Clin N Am 36 (2024) 61–72
https://doi.org/10.1016/j.coms.2023.09.007

Vascular anomalies mainly affect soft tissues and primary intraosseous vascular lesions affecting the craniofacial region are uncommon and account for less than 1% of osseous tumors.[8] Bony changes in hemangiomas were reported in only 1% of cases and were related to bony distortions such as depression of the outer cortex, nasal deviation, or orbital enlargement in the proliferative phase of hemangiomas.[8,9] Bony changes can however be present in up to 34% of vascular malformations. These changes in bone development were classified according to size, shape, and density changes. Hypertrophy and distortion were typical of lymphatic malformations. Hypoplasia and demineralization were characteristic finding in extremity venous malformations. Destructive and intraosseous changes were more commonly noted in arterial or high-flow lesions. Possible mechanisms of altered skeletal growth were postulated to include mechanical, physiologic, and developmental processes.[8]

The use of inaccurate nomenclature is even more pronounced in the case of intraosseous vascular/venous malformations.[10–16] Srinivasan and colleagues[10,11] found that all their patients found to have intraosseous venous malformation (IOVM) were all initially reported as "haemangiomas." Liberale and colleagues[16] reviewed the literature concerning vascular malformations of the bone, which had been reported as angioma, hemangioma, or hemangioendothelioma, published between January 2013 and October 2018. Clinical features, imaging, and histologic reports contained in the papers were reviewed and the diagnosis reclassified according to the 2018 ISSVA classification. Almost all the vascular anomalies presented in the reviewed papers as angiomas, hemangiomas, or hemangioendotheliomas were venous (mostly) or arteriovenous malformations. Only 8 out of 58 papers (14.7%) had an accurate diagnosis. Interestingly, all the papers reporting cavernous or capillary hemangiomas were actually venous malformations. In this article, the lesions will be described as per the recent ISSVA classifications, but the literature review will be presented with the terminology used in the relevant publications.

PATHOGENESIS

A detailed description of the pathogenesis and genetic basis of the disease is beyond the scope of this article. In brief, the identification of gene mutation(s) in each disease through the widespread use of next-generation sequencers is a clue to the understanding of the 2018 ISSVA classification. Causative genes for vascular anomalies are often found on molecules on the rat sarcoma (RAS)/mitogen-activated protein kinase kinase (MEK)/extracellular signal regulated kinase (ERK) pathway and phosphatidylinositol-4,5-bisphosphate 3-kinase catalytic subunit alpha (PIK3CA)/ak strain transforming (Akt)/mamilian target of rapamycin (mTOR) pathway.[17]

The RAS/MEK/ERK pathway, as the so-called "RASopathy," mainly causes high-flow vascular malformations, including arteriovenous malformations and vascular tumors. On the other hand, the PIK3CA/Akt/mTOR pathway, as "PIKopathy," induces slow-flow vascular malformations, such as venous or lymphatic malformations.

DIAGNOSIS

Diagnosis can often be established with a thorough history, clinical examination, and appropriate imaging.

Bone involvement can be isolated or form part of a more extensive soft tissue lesion. Most patients present with an enlarging hard lump with some reporting associated discomfort. Discoloration of the overlying skin and mucosa, pulsation, bruit, and compressibility can be present, especially when the bone involvement is associated with adjacent soft tissue involvement. Facial asymmetry, malocclusion, tooth displacement and mobility, and bleeding, including catastrophic bleeding following tooth extractions have all been reported at presentation.[8,9,11,14] The history of trauma was reported in up to 50% of patients.[11] These lesions were more common in females with a male-to-female ratio of 1:3. The age range at presentation for venous malformations was 15 to 74 years, though most presented in the fourth to sixth decades.[11] This differed from the high-flow arteriovenous malformations which presented earlier; most frequently in the third decade.[18] The duration the lesions had been present varied from 2 months to 6 years.

IMAGING
Intraosseous Venous Malformations

These demonstrate low-to-intermediate signal intensity on T1; there may be areas of sporadic internal T1-shortening at sites of hemorrhage or thrombosis.[18,19] On T2 they will demonstrate heterogeneous, high signal intensity. There is heterogenous, avid contrast enhancement, which may be delayed. Internal areas of signal void may be visible, often in a spiculated "sunburst" pattern, representing the characteristic radiating internal bony trabeculae. The sunburst pattern results from bony displacement by a network of vascular spaces, with reactive new bone formation resulting in thickened trabeculae. When these trabeculae are viewed in cross section, a "honeycomb" or "soap bubble" appearance is described. On CT, this trabecular pattern will be highlighted against a background of an expansile lucent osseous lesion, with intact cortical margins (Patients 1, 2). Phleboliths, appearing as rounded areas of signal void on MR imaging and calcification on CT, are occasionally identified, though they are considerably less frequent in IOVMs compared with their soft tissue counterparts.

Arteriovenous Malformations

CT with early arterial enhancement (CT angiography) and three-dimensional reconstruction images are quite helpful for diagnosis, follow-up, and planning of treatment.[19–21] Current technique with three-dimensional reconstruction provides information about extension of the soft-tissue arteriovenous malformation (AVM) lesion, feeding artery, exact shunting points, draining vein, and involvement of the bone. Typical CT finding of intraosseous AVMs is contrast-enhancing multiple small osteolytic lesions or a single large cavitary lesion in the medulla with or without cortical destruction (Patients 4, 5). For evaluation of the cortical changes by AVMs, CT is better than MRI.

MRI can determine and distinguish between high-flow and low-flow malformations.[19–21] Further, various imaging sequences make it easy to determine relationships to adjacent anatomic structures such as organs, muscles, nerves, and so on. The high temporal resolution of time-resolved MR angiography enables arterial, venous, and nidus localization. Intraosseous AVMs typically demonstrate signal voids in the cortex or medulla on most sequences. These flow voids are felt to be predominantly due to time-of-flight phenomena with turbulence-related rephasing also contributing to signal loss. An additional feature to differentiate high-flow lesions from low-flow lesions is the presence of enlarged feeding arteries and dilated draining veins. Gradient echo sequences show AVMs as bright, signal, serpiginous, and vascular structures (Patients 4, 5).

CT and MR Angiograms and Catheter Angiograms

CT and MR angiograms are useful in the evaluation of flow and vascularity of the lesion and for initial decisions about the likelihood of potential embolization in its management. Digitally subtracted catheter angiography is principally used when embolization is considered for the management of the lesions, rather than for purely "diagnostic" purposes (Patients 4, 5).

Histopathology and immunohistochemistry

Histopathological analysis heamatoxylin and eosin (H&E) demonstrates thin-walled vascular channels lined by flattened endothelium with scant stroma and lacking a uniform muscular layer and can be useful in differentiating hemangiomas from vascular malformations. Vascular anomalies are notoriously difficult to diagnose and classify due to overlapping histologically features and until recently lack of specific markers to distinguish these lesions. Immuno-histochemical analysis, especially glucose transporter 1 (GLUT 1) stains can provide additional certainty of diagnosis. North and colleagues[22] initially reported the utility of GLUT 1 in differentiating hemangiomas and vascular malformations and demonstrated that 97% of hemangiomas expressed GLUT 1 staining (sensitivity 95%, Specificity 100%), but none of the vascular malformations expressed GLUT 1 staining (sensitivity and specificity 100%). Other investigators have subsequently confirmed the utility of GLUT 1 stains in differentiating between these two lesions, but principally for soft tissue lesions.[23]

Srinivasan and colleagues[10,11] and Bruder and colleagues[15] reported the use of GLUT 1 in diagnosing intraosseous venous/vascular malformations and highlighted the lack of staining, similar to that seen in the soft tissue lesions.

MANAGEMENT

Management of intraosseous vascular lesions is based on the specific diagnosis and influenced by the patients' age and health, size, location, symptoms, elective/emergency presentation, team expertise, and resources.

Skull Vault Lesions

They present as a slowly enlarging mass, which can be symptomatic or picked up as an incidental finding during imaging for an unrelated problem. They account for about 0.2% of primary benign cranial tumors and 1.1% of the surgically treated cranial and spinal cavernous malformations.[24] These lesions are most frequently found in the frontal, temporal, and parietal skull.[24,25] They were more common in women (M:F—1:1.6) and most frequently presented in the fourth decade.[24]

IOVMs primarily occur within the diploic space with an expansile appearance and thinning of the overlying cortex. This appearance is best delineated with high-resolution CT imaging, which easily depicts the characteristic elements, variously described as stippled, spiculated, honeycomb, spoke wheel, or sunburst in appearance. The variable ossific density is thought reflective of osteoblastic activity from chronic and repeat hemorrhage. The imaging appearance of calvarial IOVMs with MR imaging is variable. IOVMs have strikingly hyperintense signal on T2-weighted imaging, reflecting slow-flowing blood or subacute thrombus. On T1-weighted imaging, some lesions have high signal from thrombus or fat, which may be differentiated with a fat-suppressed technique. Residual cortex has thin and hypointense signal on all MR pulse sequences, and the internal ossific spicules may be evident as internal areas of signal void. Extraosseous soft-tissue extension is possible and better discriminated on MR imaging, given its advantage in soft-tissue contrast resolution.[24]

Heckel and colleagues[25] reported expansion of the outer table with the inner table being intact in a majority of cases, with resorption of the inner table being found in larger lesions and lagging behind the changes in the outer table. Wang and colleagues[24] reported that the inner table was invaded and destroyed in the majority of patients in their series and felt because the lesions were much larger are the only intact inner table was found in the patient whose tumor was the smallest in our series (1.0 cm).

Conservative management with clinical and imaging surveillance can be an option for asymptomatic vascular malformations away from esthetically critical areas.

Lesions that are symptomatic, enlarging, and present in locations that are esthetical critical are managed by surgery. Adjuvant interventions will depend on the specific diagnosis of the lesions.

Surgery remains the mainstay of treatment for these lesions. Curettage is generally not recommended due to the risk of bleeding and incomplete excision. Complete excision outside the perimeter of these lesions is recommended to reduce the risk of bleeding and recurrence. An accurate assessment of the clinical finding and cross-sectional imaging is mandatory to determine the margins of the lesions and plan the resection.

We currently use surgical guides and intraoperative navigation to enable safe and complete excision. There were no instances of increased intraoperative bleeding in our series. Tailored reconstruction of the resultant defect is necessary to achieve excellent functional and esthetic outcomes. Titanium mesh and bone grafts are among the most frequently used reconstructive methods described in the literature.[24] Surgical guides and patient-specific implants were most frequently used in our practice.

Patient 1

A 76-year-old woman presented with a slowly enlarging swelling in the left forehead of a year's duration (**Fig. 1**A). It had more recently been associated with discomfort and she denied any previous history of trauma. A CT scan demonstrated an expansile lesion with a narrow zone of transition and a sun burst pattern of trabecular thickening radiating from the center. The inner cortex was intact (**Fig. 1**B, C).

A hemicoronal flap within the hairline (**Fig. 1**D) was raised in the subgaleal plane and a separate pericranial flap created (**Fig. 1**E). The lesion was exposed (**Fig. 1**F) and a surgical guide was placed to facilitate the planned resection margins and reconstruction (**Fig. 1**G, H). A full-thickness excision of the calvarium was carried out (**Fig. 1**I). A PEEK patient-specific implant was used to reconstruct the defect and held in place with plates (**Fig. 1**J). A folded pericranial flap (**Fig. 1**K) was placed over the implant and the wound closed in layers (**Fig. 1**L).

ORBITAL RIMS AND ZYGOMA

Zygoma and the periorbital bone are the second most common sites of intraosseous vascular malformation in the facial skeleton, following the jaw bones.[10,26] There was a female predilection (F:M—3:1), and they most frequently presented in the fourth decade. A history of trauma was elicited in 14% of patients. The lesions were described as symptomatic (pain/discomfort) in 37% of patients and 14% demonstrated ophthalmologic changes.[10,26] In frontal lesions involving the orbital rim and walls and other periorbital intraosseous lesions including those arising from the zygoma, additional factors such as orbital dystopia, proptosis, diplopia, foraminal, and fissural compression would also have to be considered when determining the need for intervention. The risk of damage to the orbital structures, and extension of the resultant defect into the nasal cavity and adjacent air sinuses will have to be carefully assessed and is likely to influence the resection and the subsequent reconstruction.

Complete surgical excision was the most frequently carried out treatment and was reported in 86% of cases. Partial excision and curettage were reported in a smaller number of patients and can be associated with an increased risk of recurrence.[10,26,27] The need to accurately recreate the premorbid orbital shape and volume in paramount to achieve excellent cosmesis and function. Intraoperative navigation will greatly help in confirming the location of the relevant and critical structures and achieving the preplanned resection of the

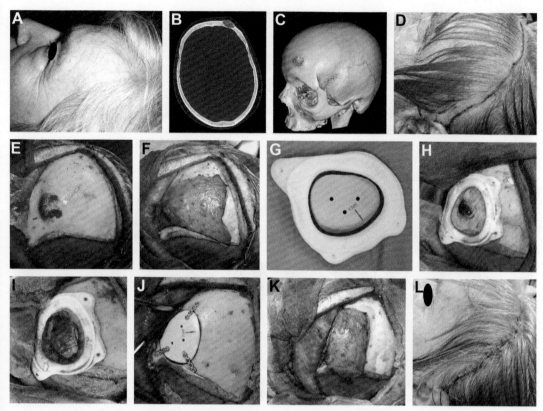

Fig. 1. Patient 1: (*A*) Prominent lesion left forehead. (*B*) Axial CT with a honey comb intradiploeic lesion, with intact inner cortex. (*C*) 3D reformatted CT. (*D*) Skin marking for hemicoronal flap. (*E*) Exposed lesion. (*F*) Pericranial flap. (*G*) Surgical guide and patient-specific PEEK implant. (*H*) Surgical guide in situ. (*I*) Defect following resection. (*J*) Patient-specific PEEK implant in situ. (*K*) Implant covered with pericranial flap. (*L*) Wound closure.

lesion. Accurate reconstruction of the defect is best achieved with patient-specific implants and surgical guides.[26] Contoured bone grafts have been the most frequently reported reconstructive method (split calvarium > iliac crest > rib) and were carried out primarily, but the need for an additional donor site (including split calvarial bone grafts), the unpredictable resorption in the postoperative period, and difficulty in recreating the complex three-dimensional anatomy of these sites consistently, makes it a less than ideal reconstructive option.[26] Although "on table" contouring of a titanium mesh can be undertaken for more "straight forward" defects, a pre-contoured implant created on stereolithographic models or computerized planning is preferred for the more complex defects. The choice of the alloplastic material is varied and will be determined by the need for intraoperative adjustments, imaging surveillance, clinician experience/preference, and resources.

Patient 2

A 46-year-old woman presented with a right supraorbital swelling of 1-month duration. A CT and MRI scan were reported as keeping with an intraosseous (hemangioma) venous malformation. The patient initially elected to pursue a "conservative" course with clinical and imaging surveillance. The lesions had continued to grow and were becoming more noticeable and symptomatic and she elected for surgery 18 months after the initial presentation (**Fig. 2**A). A CT scan confirmed a lesion in the right supraorbital rim, exhibiting sun burst pattern of trabeculae radiating from the center and extending into the orbital roof (**Fig. 2**B, C). A virtual surgical plan was undertaken to determine the extent of resection and the resultant defect was "virtually reconstructed" by mirroring the contralateral side (**Fig. 2**D). A stereolithographic model was created with the "reconstructed" defect and used to prebend a patient-specific titanium mesh (**Fig. 2**E).

A hemi coronal flap was raised in the subgaleal plane and the lesion exposed (**Fig. 2**F, G). A frontal craniotomy was performed above the lesion with the aid of intraoperative navigation. The dura was separated from the anterior skull base and orbital roof. The supraorbital nerve released from their foramen, and the periorbita was elevated from the

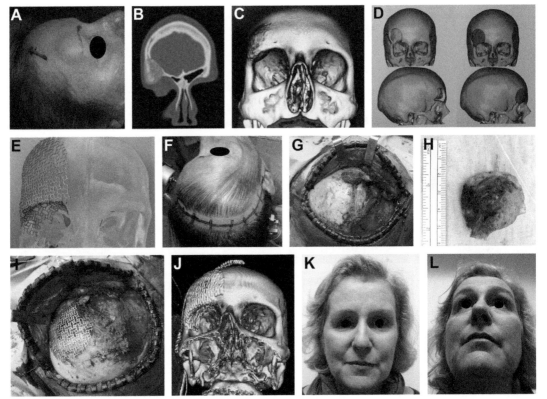

Fig. 2. Patient 2: (*A*) Prominent lesion right supraorbital region. (*B*) Coronal CT with a stipulated lesion right supraorbital rim. (*C*) 3D reformatted CT demonstrating extent of lesion. (*D*) Virtual surgical plan with defect and mirror image reconstruction. (*E*) Stereolithographic model with prebent titanium mesh. (*F*) Skin marking for hemicoronal flap. (*G*) Lesion exposed. (*H*) En bloc resection specimen. (*I*) Defect reconstructed with prebent titanium mesh. (*J*) Early 3D reformatted CT demonstrating reconstruction. (*K*) Post-op image with excellent symmetry. (*L*) Worms eye view with excellent symmetry.

orbital roof. The dura and periorbita were protected with retractors, and the bone cuts surrounding the lesion were made with the aid of image guidance. The lesion was removed en bloc (**Fig. 2**H, with no increased bleeding). The preformed titanium mesh was used to reconstruct the defect and this along with the craniotomy bone flap held in place with plates and screws (**Fig. 2**I). A postoperative CT scan (**Fig. 2**J) and clinical photos (**Fig. 2**K, L) demonstrate very satisfactory appearance.

Patient 3

A 52-year-old woman presented with a gradually enlarging swelling in the left supraorbital region of a year's duration (**Fig. 3**A). She felt it was becoming more noticeable and was having to adopt varying head position to compensate for the ptosis. A 3D reconstructed CT demonstrates the extent of the lesion and its relationship to the frontal sinus (**Fig. 3**B). A virtual surgical planning was undertaken to decide on the extent of the

resection and the subsequent reconstruction. A surgical guide was created to aid resection, and mirror image from the contralateral side was used to create the patient-specific implant (**Fig. 3**C). A hemi-coronal flap (**Fig. 3**D) was raised in the subgaleal plane and a separate pericranial flap created (**Fig. 3**E). The lesion was exposed and the surgical guide placed to aid resection (**Fig. 3**F). The defect following resection with opening into the frontal sinus is shown in **Fig. 3**G. The pericranial flap was placed in the defect to separate the implant from the sinus (**Fig. 3**H) and the implant held in place with plates (**Fig. 3**I). The wound was closed in layers (**Fig. 3**J).

Maxilla

Maxilla is among the most frequent site of a vascular malformation (AVM), second only to the mandible in the facial skeleton. There is a slight male predilection (M: F—4:3) and frequently presented in the second and third decades.[21,28] Oral (spontaneous or iatrogenic) and nasal bleeding

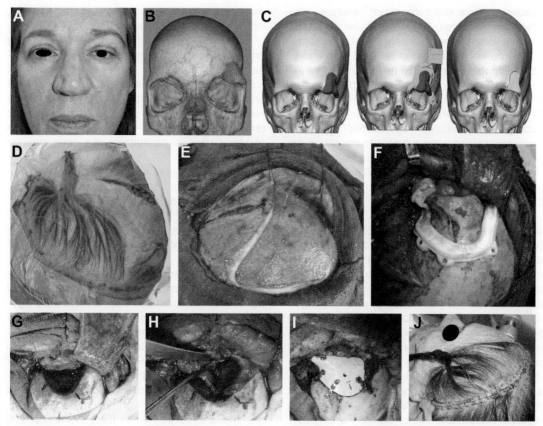

Fig. 3. Patient 3: (*A*) Prominent lesion left supraorbital rim with reduced palpebral fissure. (*B*) 3D reformatted CT demonstrating extent of lesion and relationship to frontal sinus. (*C*) Virtual surgical planning images. (*D*) Skin marking hemicoronal flap. (*E*) Pericranial flap. (*F*) Exposed lesion with surgical guide in situ. (*G*) Defect following resection with opening into the frontal sinus. (*H*) Pericranial flap in situ. (*I*) Patient-specific PEEK implant in situ. (*J*) Wound closure.

were the most common presentations of high-flow arteriovenous malformations (76%). Iatrogenic bleeding was reported in 15% of patients. Tooth displacement and mobility, mass lesion, and facial disfigurement were the other frequent modes of presentation. The lesions were most frequently located in posterior maxilla/molar region (95%).[21]

Most of the vascular malformations reported in the maxilla were high-flow arteriovenous malformations. Management of these lesions is best carried out in a multidisciplinary setting. Elective management involves a thorough workup including history and clinical examination, CT, and MRI including CT or MR angiograms to establish the diagnosis. A biopsy is avoided, so as not to precipitate torrential hemorrhage. Once the decision has been made for surgical intervention in the case of high-flow AVMs, a catheter digital subtraction angiogram is performed to accurately assess the extent of the lesion, the arterial input, and venous outflow and the feasibility of embolization. A staged procedure with embolization of the lesion followed by surgical resection within the 48 to 72 hours is recommended. Some investigators suggest that the surgical resection can be performed with external carotid artery "control" in selected cases.[5]

The surgical resection and any reconstruction need to take into account the age of the patient, extent and vascularity of the lesion, presentation (emergency/elective), potential teeth loss, and dental rehabilitation in addition to esthetic implications.

Azzolini and colleagues[29] reported an intraoral technique consisting of dental extraction, removal of the underlying vascular malformation through the alveolar process and packing with absorbable hemostatic material. This method, however, results in tooth loss. Brusati and colleagues[30] reported an alternative extraoral technique, supported by selective transarterial embolization. It consisted of curettage of the lesion through burred holes in the bone cortex, each immediately packed with oxidized cellulose to minimize bleeding. Behnia and colleagues[31] analyzed two different procedures: transmandibular curettage of AVMs versus temporary segmental ostectomy, extracorporeal malformation removal, and immediate reimplantation. Colletti and colleagues[14] described an algorithm in which preoperative embolization with NBCA was followed after 24 hours by intraoral aggressive curettage and packing with oxidized regenerated cellulose. These techniques were principally described for mandibular AVMs. Colletti reported uncontrolled bleeding when using it for a maxillary lesion and counseled caution, when using it for larger high-flow maxillary lesions.

Resection followed by free flap reconstruction has been reported for AVMs including those in the head and neck region, with good and predictable success rates.[28,32–35] There are concerns about the choice of vessels for successful anastomosis and their use following embolization. The successful use of the feeding arterial vessel, when other vessels are not available, has been described with no additional adverse risks. An increased risk of venous thrombosis has however been reported when using the enlarged draining veins.[35] The other area of debate has been the influence of free flap reconstruction in the local microenvironment of the AVM and if this leads to reduced recurrence rates. Some investigators have suggested that the physiologically normal vascular supply of the flap can potentially act as a regulating flap by suppressing residual AVM, because it seems to provide an environment that discourages microfistula opening or collateral formation,[36,37] whereas others have doubted its efficiency in this respect.[28,34,35,38]

Patient 4

A 50-year-old woman presented with an enlarging lump in her anterior maxilla, causing displacement of her teeth and discomfort (**Fig. 4**A). An MRI and CT scan reported a locally destructive mass with a sunburst appearance in the anterior maxilla with erosion of the palate, nasal septum, and teeth roots (**Fig. 4**B, C). An angiogram demonstrated a vascular lesion principally supplied by the descending palatine vessels (**Fig. 4**D). Following preoperative embolization, the lesion was access with a modified Weber–Fergusson and upper vestibular incisions and the lesion margins exposed, preserving the palatal mucosa (**Fig. 4**E, F). The pre-planned bone cuts were made with a Sonopet (**Fig. 4**G–I) and the lesion removed en bloc with no increased bleeding (**Fig. 4**J, K). The defect was reconstructed with a myo-osseous scapula tip free flap (**Fig. 4**L–N) Late postoperative result

demonstrated very satisfactory esthetic outcome, including dental rehabilitation (**Fig. 4**O–R).

The term of "nidus" (breeding place, breeding ground) is a clinical term created by the radiologists to describe the bundle/cluster of small sized AV connections/fistulae, filled with contrast on arteriography and other tests. This is NOT a histologic term, nor an anatomic/pathologic term but a descriptive term of a conglomerate of blood vessels constituting the arteriovenous malformation.

A "nidus" is almost always present in an extra-truncular lesion and appears as a net of dysplastic pulsating, tortuous vessels between the artery and vein. The "nidus" of the lesion retains its "diffuse, multiple small fistulous" condition in contrast to the truncular lesion, which often have large individual arteriovenous fistulas.

Occlusion or removal of the arteriovenous malformations "nidus" should be the main goal of treatment. Transarterial coil, embolization, or ligation of feeding arteries, where the nidus is left intact, are incorrect approaches and may result in proliferation of the lesion. Furthermore, such procedures would prevent future endovascular access to the lesions via the arterial route.

Embolization as the "sole" modality of treatment has been described for high-flow maxilla-mandibular AVMs especially when there is minimal soft tissue extension.[39] Maxillary lesions were more frequently associated with soft tissue involvement and required increased number of treatments, with "cure" rates approaching 46% (vs 70% mandible). Rodesh and colleagues[40] reported cure rates of 34% and stability in 100% of patients with embolization via the transarterial and direct intraosseous puncture routes, using poly vinyl alcohol and n-butyl cyanoacrylate (n-BCA).

Endovascular management is however the treatment of choice for patients presenting as an emergency with significant bleeding, which cannot be controlled with local measures such as packing. Churojana and colleagues[41] reported five patients presenting with life-threatening bleeding who were managed with super-selective embolization and direct transosseous puncture, using n-BCA. Su and colleagues[42] reported 12 patients with hemorrhagic arteriovenous malformation who were managed successfully with transarterial and direct puncture embolization with absolute ethanol aided with the use of coils.

Common embolic agents for AVM treatment include ethanol, n-BCA glue, Onyx (Microtherapeutics, Inc, Irvine, CA), and coils. However, no consensus exists regarding the most effective treatment, and each agent has its own pros and cons.

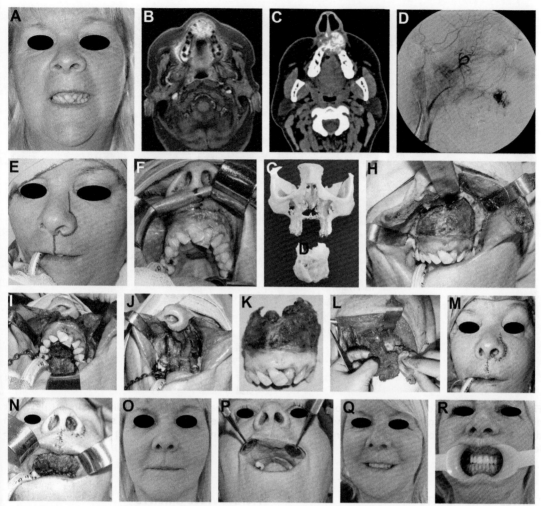

Fig. 4. Patient 4: (*A*) Mass lesion anterior maxilla with displaced teeth. (*B*) MRI image with high signal lesion in the anterior maxilla. (*C*) Axial CT with locally destructive lesion anterior maxilla. (*D*) Digital subtraction angiogram demonstrating vascular lesion anterior maxilla. (*E*) Skin marking for planned access. (*F*) Lesion with markings for mucosal incisions. (*G*) Stereolithographic mode with planned surgical resection. (*H*) Labial bone cuts. (*I*) Preserved palatal mucosa and palatal bone cuts. (*J*) Defect following resection. (*K*) En bloc resection specimen. (*L*) Myo-osseus scapula tip free flap. (*M*) Wound closure. (*N*) Intraoral appearance. (*O*) Post-op external appearance. (*P*) Post-op intraoral appearance. (*Q*) Dentures in situ. (*R*) Dentures in situ.

Lilje and colleagues in a systematic review reported that the data on interventional therapy for the management of extracranial arteriovenous malforamtions lacked consistency and quality and called for standardized reporting.[43]

Patient 5

A 10-year-old girl with a known high-flow maxillomandibular arteriovenous malformation presented as an emergency with spontaneous torrential oral bleeding from her left maxilla. Previous CT and MRI demonstrate the extent of the lesion (**Fig. 5**A–C). The lesion was principally centered on the posterior maxilla with extension into the infratemporal and pterygopalatine fossa. The bleeding was controlled with digital gauze pressure, tranexamic acid, and the patient stabilized with fluid and blood resuscitation. A catheter digital subtraction angiogram confirmed the extent of the lesion and the feeding vessels including the enlarged maxillary artery and draining veins (**Fig. 5**D). The lesion was embolized with Squid (Balt, Irvine, CA) and PHIL (Precipitating hydrophobic injectable liquid, Microvention, CA) supplemented with coils (**Fig. 5**E). She made an uneventful recovery, with no further bleeding episodes and remains under close surveillance.

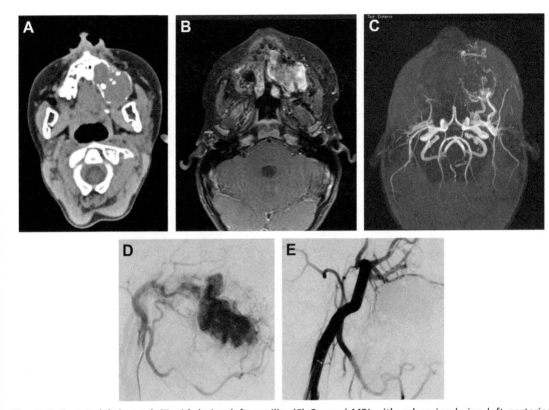

Fig. 5. Patient 5: (*A*) Coronal CT with lesion left maxilla. (*B*) Coronal MRI with enhancing lesion left posterior maxilla. (*C*) Time-of-flight MR image demonstrating a nidus of the lesion. (*D*) Digital subtraction angiogram demonstrating the vascularity of the lesion. (*E*) Post-embolization image demonstrating good occlusion of the lesion.

CLINICS CARE POINTS

- Cross-sectional imaging with CT/MR angiograms are helpful in diagnosing high-flow arteriovenous malformations.
- Catheter digital subtraction angiograms should be reserved for lesions considered for intervention rather than diagnosis.
- Emergency control of bleeding can include external pressure and packing, temporary vascular clamps and slings following exposure of the vessels or intra-arterial balloon occlusion.
- Transarterial coil, embolization, or ligation of feeding arteries, where the nidus is left intact, are incorrect approaches and may result in proliferation of the lesion.
- Such procedures also prevent future endovascular access to the lesions via the arterial route.

ACKNOWLEDGMENTS

The author would like to acknowledge the ongoing support of his consultant colleagues Mr Sanjay Sharma, Mr Nigel Horlock, Mr Nijaguna Mathad, Mr Emad Shenouda, Dr Adam Ditchfield and Dr Ana Narata, who have helped in the management of these and other patients with vascular anomalies.

REFERENCES

1. Ethunandan M, Mellor TK. Haemangiomas and vascular malformations of the maxillofacial region-A review. Br J Oral Maxillofac Surg 2006;44: 263–72.
2. Mulliken JB, Glowacki J. Hemangiomas and vascular malformations in infants and children: a classification based on endothelial characteristics. Plast Reconstr Surg 1982;69:412–22.
3. Jackson IT, Carreno R, Potparic Z, et al. Hemangiomas, vascular malformations, and lymphovenous malformations: classification and methods of treatment. Plast Reconstr Surg 1993;91:1216–30.

4. ISSVA Classification of Vascular Anomalies ©2018 International Society for the Study of Vascular Anomalies. Available at: issva.org/classification. Accessed June 12, 2023.

5. Nair SC, Spencer NJ, Nayak KP, et al. Surgical management of vascular lesions of the head and neck: a review of 115 cases. Int J Oral Maxillofac Surg 2011; 40:577–83.

6. Bolt JW, Raphael MF, Pasmans SG, et al. Discrepancies in Initial Clinical and Radiological Diagnoses of Vascular Malformations and the Role of the ISSVA Classification. J Vascular Anomalies 2023;4(1):e057.

7. Hassanein AH, Mulliken JB, Fishman SJ, et al. Evaluation of terminology for vascular anomalies in current literature. Plast Reconstr Surg 2011;127: 347–51.

8. Boyd JB, Mulliken JB, Kaban LB, et al. Skeletal changes associated with vascular malformations. Plast Reconstr Surg 1984;74:789.

9. Williams HB. Facial bone changes with vascular tumors in children. Plast Reconstr Surg 1979;63:309.

10. Srinivasan B, Ethunandan M, Van der Horst C, et al. Intra-osseous "haemangioma" of the zygoma: more appropriately termed a venous malformation. Int J Oral Maxillofac Surg 2009;38:1066–70.

11. Srinivasan B, Chan E, Mellor T, et al. Intra osseous venous malformation of the craniofacial regions: diagnosis and management. Br J Oral Maxillofac Surg 2019;57:1143–7.

12. Kadlub N, Dainese L, Coulomb L, et al. Intra osseous haemangioma: semantic and medical confusion. Int J Oral Maxillofac Surg 2015;44:718–24.

13. Werdich XQ, Jackobiec FA, Curtin HD, et al. A clinical, radiologic and immunopathologic study of five periorbital intra osseous cavernous vascular malformations. Am J Ophthalmol 2014;158:816–26.

14. Colletti G, Frigerio A, Giovanditto F, et al. Surgical treatment of vascular malformations of the facial bones. J Oral Maxillofac Surg 2014;72:1326.e1-18.

15. Bruder E, Perez-Atayde AR, Jundt G, et al. Vascular lesions of bone in children, adolescents and young adults. A clinicopathologic reappraisal and application of the ISSVA classification. Virchows Arch 2009; 454:161–79.

16. Liberale C, Rozell-Shannon L, Moneghini L, et al. Stop calling me cavernous hemangioma! A literature review on misdiagnosed bony vascular anomalies. J Investig Surg 2022;35:141–50.

17. Kunimoto K, Yamamoto Y, Jinnin M. ISSVA Classification of Vascular Anomalies and Molecular Biology. Int J Mol Sci 2022;23:2358.

18. Strauss SB, Steinklein JM, Phillips CD, et al. Intra-osseous venous malformations of the head and neck. Am J Neuroradiol 2022;43(8):1090–8.

19. Griauzde J, Srinivasan A. Imaging of vascular lesions of the head and neck. Radiol Clin North Am 2015;53(1):197–213.

20. So YS, Park KB. Special Consideration for Intraosseous Arteriovenous Malformations. Semin Intervent Radiol 2017 Sep;34(3):272–9.

21. Li X, Su L, Wang D, et al. Clinical and imaging features of intraosseous arteriovenous malformations in jaws: a 15-year experience of single centre. Sci Rep 2020;10:12046.

22. North PE, Waner M, Mizeracki, et al. GLUT 1: a newly discovered immunohistochemical marker for juvenile hemangiomas. Hum Pathol 2000;31:11–22.

23. Leon-Villapalos J, Wolfe K, Kangesu L. GLUT 1: an extra diagnostic tool to differentiate between haemangiomas and vascular malformations. Br J Plast Surg 2005;58:348–52.

24. Wang C, Zhang D, Wang S, et al. Intraosseous cavernous malformations of the skull: Clinical characteristics and long-term surgical outcomes. Neurosurg Rev 2020;43:231–9.

25. Heckl S, Aschoff A, Kunze S. Cavernomas of the skull: review of the literature 1975–2000. Neurosurg Rev 2002;25(1–2):56–62.

26. Conde RA, Cuéllar CA, Escobar JIS, et al. Intraosseous venous malformation of the zygomatic Bone: Comparison between virtual surgical planning and standard surgery with review of the literature. J Clin Med 2012;10:4565.

27. Cheng NC, Lai DR, Hsie MH, et al. Intaosseous haemagiomas of the facial bone. Plast Reconstr Surg 2006;117:2366–72.

28. Kohout MP, Hansen M, Pribaz JJ, et al. Arteriovenous malformations of the head and neck: Natural history and management. Plast Reconstr Surg 1998;102:643–54.

29. Azzolini A, Bertani A, Riberti C. Superselective embolization and immediate surgical treatment: Our present approach to treatment of large vascular hemangiomas of the face. Ann Plast Surg 1982;9:42.

30. Brusati R, Galioto S, Biglioli F, et al. Conservative treatment of arteriovenous malformations of the mandible. Int J Oral Maxillofac Surg 2001;30:397.

31. Behnia H, Ghodoosi I, Motamedi MH, et al. Treatment of arteriovenous malformations: Assessment of 2 techniques—Transmandibular curettage versus resection and immediate replantation. J Oral Maxillofac Sur 2008;66:2557.

32. Koshima I, Nanba Y, Tsutsui T, et al. Free perforator flap for the treatment of defects after resection of huge arteriovenous malformations in the head and neck region. Ann Plast Surg 2003;51:194–9.

33. Yamamoto Y, Ohura T, Minakawa H, et al. Experience with arteriovenous malformations treated with flap coverage. Plast Reconstr Surg 1994;94:476–82.

34. Hartzell LD, Stack BC Jr, Yuen J, et al. Free tissue reconstruction following excision of head and neck arteriovenous malformations. Arch Facial Plast Surg 2009;11:171–7.

35. Fujiki M, Ozaki M, Iwashina Y, et al. Clinical outcomes and recipient vessel selection for free flap transfer following arteriovenous malformation resection. J Plast Surg Hand Surg 2018;53:56–9.

36. Dompmartin A, Labbe D, Barrellier MT, et al. Use of a regulating flap in the treatment of a large arteriovenous malformation. Br J Plast Surg 1998;51:561–3.

37. Tark KC, Chung S. Histological change of arteriovenous malformations of the face and scalp after free flap transfer. Plast Reconstr Surg 2000;106:87–93.

38. Liu AS, Mulliken JB, Zurakowski D, et al. Extracranial arteriovenous malformations: natural progression and recurrence after treatment. Plast Reconstr Surg 2010;125:1185–94.

39. Persky MS, Yoo HJ, Berenstein A. Management of vascular malformations of the mandible and maxilla. Laryngoscope 2003;113:1885–92.

40. Rodesch G, Soupre V, Varquez MP, et al. Arteriovenous malformations of the dental arcades. The place of endovascular therapy: results in 12 cases are presented. J Cranio-Maxillo-Fac Surg 1998;26:306–13.

41. Churojana A, Khumtong R, Songsaeng D, et al. Life-threatening arteriovenous malformation of the maxilliomandibular region and treatment outcomes. Intervent Neuroradiol 2012;18:49–59.

42. Su L, Wang D, Han Y, et al. Salvage treatment of hemorrhagic arteriovenous malformations in jaws. J Cranio-Maxillo-Fac Surg 2015;43:1082–7.

43. Lilje D, Wiesmann M, Hasan D, et al. Interventional therapy of extracranial arteriovenous malformations of the head and neck – A systematic review. PLoS One 2022;17(7):e0268809.

Airway Considerations in Vascular Lesions

Kaylee R. Purpura, MD[a],*, Joshua S. Schindler, MD[b]

KEYWORDS

- Difficult airway management • Airway obstruction • Flexible fiberoptic laryngoscopy
- Awake intubation • Laser precautions

KEY POINTS

- A flexible fiberoptic laryngoscopy should be performed on patients with vascular anomalies to evaluate lesions of the upper aerodigestive tract to understand the full extent of 1 or more lesions.
- Anesthesia and otolaryngology consults should be considered preoperatively for assistance with management of a difficult airway.
- Multiple backup plans should be discussed if intubation is anticipated to be difficult in patients with head and neck vascular anomalies, including alternative intubation methods and awake procedures.
- Edema and hemorrhage should be expected complications following treatment, and a plan for the airway at the end of the procedure should be discussed.
- Laser precautions should be taken when a laser is used for treatment of a vascular anomaly because the head and neck is at higher risk of complications.

INTRODUCTION

Vascular anomalies are congenital lesions that can be broadly classified as vascular tumors and vascular malformations. The most common type of vascular tumors are infantile hemangiomas.[1,2] Vascular malformations are broadly classified by the type of vessel involved,[1,3] which includes capillary, venous, lymphatic, and arteriovenous malformations.[2–4] Infantile hemangiomas have 3 characteristic phases, including proliferation, plateau, and eventual involution.[3] Vascular malformations are persistent and tend to increase in size with time.[3,4] It is important to correctly identify these lesions because they behave differently, as does their treatment.[1]

Head and neck vascular lesions often require a multidisciplinary approach for treatment and special considerations for management of the airway.[3] More than half of vascular lesions occur in the head and neck,[5] and about 40% of venous malformations are seen in the head and neck.[4–6] Infantile hemangiomas are the most common vascular tumor to involve the airway,[3] and about 60% involve the head and neck.[2] About 73% of patients with head and neck lymphatic malformations will have involvement of the upper aerodigestive tract, most commonly including the tongue, oropharynx, and supraglottis. Multiple sites may be diffusely involved as well[3] and lead to airway obstruction.

Airway Involvement

All of the different types of vascular lesions can affect the airway and disrupt the function of the upper aerodigestive tract,[7] which includes the nasopharynx, oral cavity, oropharynx, supraglottis, glottis, subglottis, hypopharynx, and trachea.[3] Vascular anomalies in these areas can lead to functional complications with speech, mastication, deglutition, and airway obstruction.[1,3,5] These lesions are most challenging when function is affected, especially the airway.[8] Airway obstruction can manifest in several ways, including stridor,

[a] Department of Otolaryngology - Head and Neck Surgery, MedStar Georgetown University Hospital, 3800 Reservoir Road NW, Washington, DC 20007, USA; [b] Department of Otolaryngology–Head and Neck Surgery, Oregon Health and Science University, 3181 Southwest Sam Jackson Park Road, Portland, OR 97239, USA
* Corresponding author.
E-mail address: kayleepurpura@gmail.com

Oral Maxillofacial Surg Clin N Am 36 (2024) 73–80
https://doi.org/10.1016/j.coms.2023.09.002

which is a high-pitched noise associated with obstruction at the level of the glottis or subglottis, stertor, which indicates obstruction above the glottis within the nasopharynx or oropharynx, increased work of breathing, tachypnea, retractions, and respiratory failure.[1]

FLEXIBLE FIBEROPTIC LARYNGOSCOPY

Patients with vascular lesions of the head and neck should have a flexible fiberoptic laryngoscopy performed prior to any planned interventions to evaluate the whole upper aerodigestive tract and lesions that may not be seen externally that could cause airway obstruction. A thorough flexible fiberoptic evaluation should be performed by a provider that routinely performs these examinations. It is better tolerated by patients if the nasal cavities are anesthetized with a topical anesthetic and a nasal decongestant to help constrict the inferior turbinates to allow for easier passage of the fiberoptic scope through the nasal cavities. Allowing 5 to 10 minutes for the medication to take effect is helpful to increase patient tolerance. Bilateral nasal cavities should be evaluated to the nasopharynx. Palate elevation should be documented along with any evidence of velopharyngeal insufficiency as a result of a vascular lesion. **Fig. 1** shows an image from a flexible fiberoptic laryngoscopy of a patient with a venous malformation of the nasopharynx that extends to the posterior pharyngeal wall and the base of the tongue. To evaluate the oropharynx, the patient should stick out their tongue to evaluate tongue protrusion

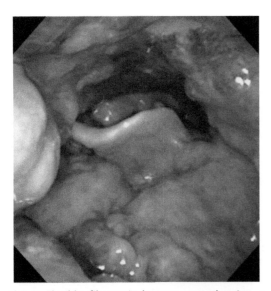

Fig. 1. Flexible fiberoptic laryngoscopy showing a venous malformation involving the posterior pharyngeal wall, post cricoid area, and base of the tongue.

and lesions of the base of the tongue, vallecula, and epiglottis. Having the patient cough to clear any secretions and then swallow will allow for evaluation of their swallowing and movement of the epiglottis. **Fig. 2** shows a venous malformation that involves the epiglottis, vallecula, and left hypopharynx. To evaluate the hypopharynx, the patient should hold their breath and puff up their cheeks. Voicing tasks, such as phonating "eee", alternating between a sniff and an "e", and counting to 10 will allow for evaluation of the movement of the bilateral arytenoid cartilages and true vocal folds along with alteration of the movement by an obstructive lesion. During laryngoscopy, care should be taken to prevent traumatizing lesions[1] so as not to cause bleeding or dynamic changes from coughing or gagging. The size and extent of any lesions along with the involved structures, including proximity to the airway,[9] and alteration of function should be well-documented.[1]

TREATMENT OPTIONS

The planned intervention for these lesions depends on correctly identifying the type of lesion, extent and depth of the lesion, and concern for airway obstruction,[2,3] all of which can be evaluated on physical examination and flexible fiberoptic laryngoscopy. The management is also dependent on the experience and preference of the treating physicians in a multidisciplinary team.[2] If a patient has laryngeal involvement from a vascular anomaly, then they should undergo a direct microlaryngoscopy for full evaluation of the disease to determine potential treatment options.[3]

There are several options for the treatment of vascular lesions, but they are challenging to treat as patient results vary widely.[4] The main forms of treatment include medical management, sclerotherapy, surgical resection,[4] and laser therapy, or a combination of therapies.[10] Prior to any procedure, it is critical to fully evaluate the patient, their symptoms, and understand the behavior of the lesion being treated.

- Venous malformations are compressible lesions that can fluctuate in size with Valsalva, dependent patient positioning,[3] and increased venous pressure.[4] A patient without airway obstruction and normal respiration in a seated position may develop airway obstruction when recumbent. Up to 70% of patients with head and neck cutaneous venous malformations have involvement of the airway. All patients with cutaneous venous malformation lesions should have a flexible fiberoptic laryngoscopy to evaluate the nasopharynx, oropharynx, and

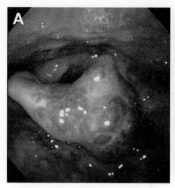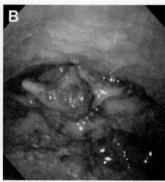

Fig. 2. Flexible fiberoptic laryngoscopy showing a venous malformation of the epiglottis (*A*) that extends along the lingual surface to the vallecula and the left hypopharynx (*B*).

glottis. Venous malformations may involve any part of the upper aerodigestive tract and can have bleeding even with minor manipulation or trauma. Patients with laryngeal involvement may have dysphonia, obstructive sleep apnea (47%–85% of patients), and upper airway obstruction, especially when lying flat.[3]

- Lymphatic malformations may change in size with upper respiratory infections due to inflammation or develop a superimposed infection that can cause airway obstruction and difficulty breathing.[11] These lesions can be microcystic, macrocytic, or mixed. Lesions involving multiple sites may require a tracheostomy for treatment due to the anticipated edema that will result from surgery or sclerotherapy.[3] Medical management of the edema with steroids may be helpful in decreasing the swelling after treatment.[3,10] It should be considered to place a drain after a surgical procedure to allow for drainage of any fluid that may persist and decrease the risk of a seroma.[10]

Edema should be anticipated and expected after surgical, sclerotherapy, or laser treatment of venous and lymphatic malformations because the malformations are draining tissues of the head and neck and altering the drainage pattern can lead to swelling. Lymphatic drainage of other sites, such as the oral cavity or oropharynx, can be altered and lead to airway obstruction as well. Anticipation of these complications will help with the postoperative plan, which may be to perform a tracheostomy or keep a patient intubated for a prolonged period of time to allow resolution of the edema or bleeding.[4]

MANAGEMENT OF A DIFFICULT AIRWAY

The basic principles of airway management apply when considering management of head and neck vascular lesions.[1] It is critical to consider how a

procedure will affect and alter the airway in order to manage complications.[9] Airway obstruction can occur before, during, or after treatment of a vascular anomaly. Recognizing that a patient may have a difficult airway due to the extent and location of a vascular lesion is key to appropriately managing the airway during treatment, whether that is laser, surgical, or sclerotherapy treatment. Being unprepared for a difficult airway is the main cause of errors in the algorithm for difficult intubation.[12] In 2022, the American Society of Anesthesiologists updated the practice guidelines for the management of the difficult airway.[13] The difficult airway algorithm is shown in **Fig. 3**, and can be used as a reference and guide for decision-making for a patient that is anticipated to have a difficult airway for intubation. A multidisciplinary approach should be taken with consultation of anesthesia and otolaryngology for assistance with the management of a possible difficult airway and to prepare a team to manage an anticipated difficult intubation and extubation.

History and Physical Examination

A history and physical examination of the airway should be performed prior to induction of anesthesia and manipulation of the airway.[12] Important history to obtain is previously being difficult to intubate, snoring or a history of obstructive sleep apnea, diabetes, and findings on diagnostic imaging, such as upper aerodigestive masses.[13] Clinical characteristics of the patient should be noted as well, including their age, sex, height, weight,[13] body mass index, and neck circumference. The physical examination is important to detect physical features that may indicate that the patient will have a difficult airway (**Box 1**).[12]

Intubation Setting

The setting for the procedure needs to be carefully considered as well. If a procedure is performed on

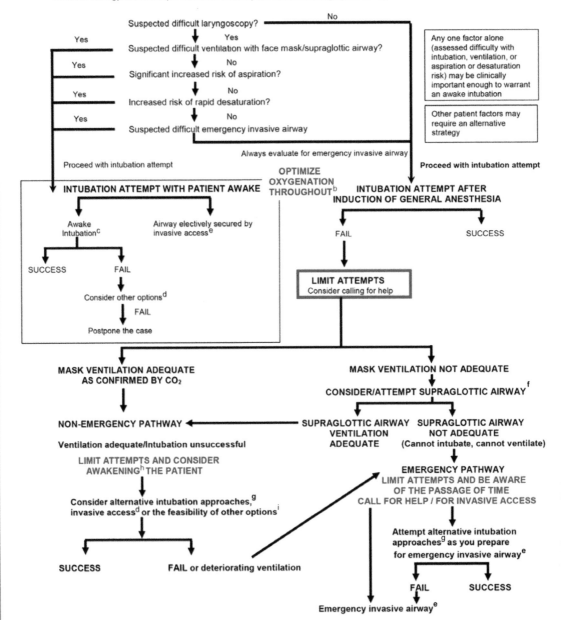

Fig. 3. The American Society of Anesthesiologists' difficult airway algorithm for adult patients. [a]The airway manager's choice of airway strategy and techniques should be based on their previous experience; available resources, including equipment, availability and competency of help; and the context in which airway management will occur. [b]Low- or high-flow nasal cannula, head elevated position throughout procedure. Noninvasive ventilation during preoxygenation. [c]Awake intubation techniques include flexible bronchoscope, videolaryngoscopy, direct laryngoscopy, combined techniques, and retrograde wire-aided intubation. [d]Other options include, but are not limited to, alternative awake technique, awake elective invasive airway, alternative anesthetic techniques, induction of anesthesia (if unstable or cannot be postponed) with preparations for emergency invasive airway and post-poning the case without attempting the above options. [e]Invasive airway techniques include surgical cricothyrotomy, needle cricothyrotomy with a pressure-regulated device, large-bore cannula cricothyrotomy, or surgical tracheostomy. Elective invasive airway techniques include the above and retrograde wire–guided intubation and percutaneous tracheostomy. Also consider rigid bronchoscopy and ECMO.

Box 1
Physical examination predictors of difficult intubation

- Interincisor distance<3 cm
- Mallampati score>3
- Thyromental distance<3 finger breadths
- Increased neck circumference
- Decreased neck range of motion, especially poor neck extension

Adapted from O'Dell K. Predictors of difficult intubation and the otolaryngology perioperative consult. Anesthesiology Clinics. 2015;33(2):279-290; with permission.

Box 2
Predictors of difficult face mask ventilation

- Obesity/high body mass index (>26 kg/m^2)[14]
- Older age (>55 years)[14]
- Male gender
- Limited mandibular protrusion
- Decreased thyromental distance
- Presence of a beard
- Edentulous
- History of snoring

Adapted from O'Dell K. Predictors of difficult intubation and the otolaryngology perioperative consult. Anesthesiology Clinics. 2015;33(2):279-290; with permission.

---

an awake patient, then the treating team needs to be prepared for possible intubation depending on how the lesion responds to the treatment. This may be more difficult if there is significant edema or bleeding. An emergent tracheostomy may be necessary if the patient cannot be endotracheally intubated.[9] This would not be feasible in an office setting or an interventional radiology suite. Any patient that may have a difficult intubation should have the procedure performed in the operating room in a more controlled setting where more airway equipment is available if needed.

Intubation Planning

The plan for intubation is dependent on many factors including most importantly the location, type, and size of the vascular anomaly but also the comfort and expertise of the clinician team performing the intubation method. An individualized plan should be created for the patient based on the specific scenario and planned treatment.[12] The ability to mask ventilate a patient should be carefully considered as this is important for pre-oxygenation as well as a rescue approach if a patient is difficult to intubate (**Box 2**). If there is a concern about the ability to mask ventilate, then confirmation of adequate ventilation using a face mask should be performed during

induction of anesthesia but before paralytic agents are given as the patient is then no longer able to spontaneously ventilate.

Maintaining oxygenation and ventilation are the goals of airway management, and repeatedly performing ineffective methods should be avoided.[14] It is important to determine if a traditional transoral intubation under general anesthesia is a safe option, and if not, then the plan should be discussed as a team and multiple backup options should be considered. Debriefing with the entire team increases the likelihood of an effective response by all members if tracheal intubation is unsuccessful.[12,15]

Alternatives to Direct Laryngoscopy

Alternative approaches for laryngoscopy may include video-assisted devices such as the GlideScope, placing a laryngeal mask airway, direct laryngoscopy with rigid laryngoscopes such as a Dedo laryngoscope or anterior commissure laryngoscope, awake nasal flexible fiberoptic intubation, an awake tracheostomy,[12] or aborting the procedure and awakening the patient if it is safe to do so for an elective procedure.

---

[f]Consideration of size, design, positioning, and first *versus* second generation supraglottic airways may improve the ability to ventilate. [g]Alternative difficult intubation approaches include but are not limited to video-assisted laryngoscopy, alternative laryngoscope blades, combined techniques, intubating supraglottic airway (with or without flexible bronchoscopic guidance), flexible bronchoscopy, introducer, and lighted stylet or lightwand. Adjuncts that may be employed during intubation attempts include tracheal tube introducers, rigid stylets, intubating stylets, or tube changers and external laryngeal manipulation. [h]Includes postponing the case or postponing the intubation and returning with appropriate resources (eg, *personnel*, equipment, patient preparation, awake intubation). [i]Other options include, but are not limited to proceeding with procedure utilizing face mask or supraglottic airway ventilation. Pursuit of these options usually implies that ventilation will not be problematic. (*From* Apfelbaum JL, Hagberg CA, Connis RT, et al. 2022 American Society of Anesthesiologists Practice Guidelines for management of the difficult airway. Anesthesiology. 2021;136(1):31-81; with permission.)

- Videolaryngoscopes can be helpful to obtain visualization of the larynx especially in patients with limited neck movement.[12] It is a useful, alternative tool to traditional laryngoscopy that can be successful if direct laryngoscopy with a Macintosh or a Miller blade fails.
- Rigid direct laryngoscopy is a tool typically used by otolaryngologists that is helpful when other forms of direct laryngoscopy have failed. With the Dedo laryngoscope, the whole glottis is able to be visualized, and the anterior commissure laryngoscope is meant to provide a view of the anterior commissure. The anterior commissure scope is able to accommodate a 5.0 millimeters cuffed endotracheal tube or smaller, whereas a larger endotracheal tube is able to be passed through the Dedo laryngoscope.[12] Rigid direct laryngoscopy is helpful to intubate patients with fixed lesions of the glottis or subglottis.

Awake Procedure Options

Patients that already have some level of airway obstruction prior to a procedure should be considered to have an awake procedure, including awake fiberoptic intubation or tracheostomy, performed as it will allow them to continue to breath spontaneously[12] with supplemental oxygen if needed. Depending on the site of the obstruction, their respiratory status could worsen with the induction of anesthesia and laying the patient flat for intubation as they could be difficult to ventilate with a face mask.

Indications for awake fiberoptic intubation include trismus, a mass or edema of the supraglottis, and known to be difficult to mask ventilate. Awake fiberoptic intubation is not a good option for firm or fixed lesions, lesions completely obstructing the glottis, or lesions that are actively bleeding and obscure visualization with the fiberoptic scope.[12]

Awake tracheostomy is an option when there is obstruction of the glottis[12] whether from a lesion at the level of the glottis or supraglottic edema that leads to poor visualization of the glottis. The patient must also be able to cooperate for the procedure to be able to safely secure the airway. A tracheostomy may be difficult due to many patient factors though, including limited neck extension leading to poor access to the anterior neck, difficult to palpate landmarks due to previous radiation or obesity, and displacement of the airway due to a tumor or lesion (**Box 3**).[12]

Cricothyrotomy is typically a last resort and is an emergent option for airway management if other techniques have failed[15] and the patient is

---

| **Box 3** |
| **Predictors of a difficult tracheostomy** |

- Thick/obese neck
- Neck radiation
- Overlying disorder (tumor, infection)
- Displaced airway
- Fixed cervical spine flexion deformity
- Pediatric patient

From O'Dell K. Predictors of difficult intubation and the otolaryngology perioperative consult. Anesthesiology Clinics. 2015;33(2):279-290; with permission.

---

unstable for further intubation attempts. This can be a difficult procedure to perform due to the urgent nature of the procedure. Patient factors can also make it a difficult procedure, such as poorly identifiable laryngeal landmarks in a patient with a large or thick neck, shifted airway, or overlying pathology, such as a vascular anomaly, mass, inflammation, or radiation changes.[15]

Management of Lesions Based on Location

Considering the location of the vascular lesion and the level of obstruction can aid in determining the airway plan for intubating a patient for a procedure.

- A lesion that leads to obstruction of the oral cavity, such as a large lesion involving the tongue or the floor of the mouth, may exclude transoral intubation as an option. An awake nasal flexible fiberoptic intubation with the patient in an upright position to prevent the tongue from falling back[12] could be a safer option as long as the patient is appropriately counseled and anticipated to be able to tolerate the procedure.
- Lesions of the supraglottis can cause airway obstruction when the patient is laid flat for intubation and make mask ventilation difficult. These lesions may also obstruct a view of the glottis with direct laryngoscopy. An awake nasal flexible fiberoptic intubation may be a better option for these patients as well. If a view of the glottis is not well-obtained with a flexible fiberoptic examination, then an awake tracheostomy should be considered.[12]
- Lesions that involve the glottis or subglottis are better managed with a direct line of site of the glottis either with standard intubation or with rigid direct laryngoscopy if that is not an option. Direct visualization of the glottis allows for application of pressure by using a stylet or rigid telescope to advance an

A

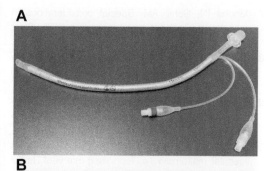

B

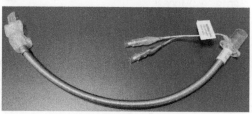

Fig. 4. Laser-safe endotracheal tubes. (*A*) Tenax laser-safe 6.0 mm endotracheal tube. (*B*) Medtronic laser-safe 6.0 mm endotracheal tube.

> **Box 4**
> **Laser precautions**
>
> - Patient and procedure precautions
>   - Use a laser-safe endotracheal tube
>   - Decrease Fio_2 to <30%
>   - Extra saline or water on the operating field
>   - Cover the patient's eyes with wet eye pads
>   - Cover the patient's face with wet towels
> - Operating room precautions
>   - Know location of the closest fire extinguisher
>   - Cover the operating room windows
>   - "Laser in use" signage on all doors
>   - Appropriate laser safety eyewear for all in the room
>   - Laser-safety operator present for the procedure

endotracheal tube past a lesion. If intubation is not feasible, then an awake tracheostomy may need to be performed.[12]

OTHER CONSIDERATIONS
Laser Precautions

Another consideration for procedures being performed with laser treatments is laser safety. Procedures on the upper aerodigestive tract have a higher risk for possible fires and mucosal burns. It is important to communicate with the anesthesia team prior to performing laser treatments and to use a laser-safe endotracheal tube, such as the Tenax Endotracheal Tube (**Fig. 4**A) or a Medtronic Shiley Laser Oral Endotracheal Tube (**Fig. 4**B). The Tenax tube is wrapped in aluminum with an outer silicone sheath,[16] and the Medtronic tube is stainless steel. Other precautions should be taken as listed in **Box 4**.

PLANNING FOR EXTUBATION

The plan for extubation at the end of a procedure also needs to be discussed as a coordinated approach with goal of determining the safest strategy to try to prevent the need for re-intubation. The setting, whether in the operating room or in the intensive care unit, and timing of extubation, whether at the end of the procedure or several days after the procedure, should be discussed.[12] Keeping the patient intubated for 48 to 72 hours can allow for edema to decrease prior to

extubation. Having to urgently re-intubate a patient should be avoided if possible because it could be more difficult due to alteration of the anatomy from the procedure, edema, or bleeding.

SUMMARY

Vascular anomalies of the head and neck can have cutaneous involvement and commonly mucosal involvement of the upper aerodigestive tract, which can lead to obstruction of the airway. It can be very difficult to intubate patients with vascular anomalies, and a coordinated approach with multiple specialties should be taken to ensure safe management of the airway. Once a patient has been identified as having a difficult airway and being difficult to intubate, it should be added to their problem list in their medical record.[12] Effective communication is the key to successful intubation and extubation.

CLINICS CARE POINTS

- When considering a surgical procedure on a patient with a vascular lesion of the head and neck, the difficult airway algorithm from the American Society of Anesthesiologists can be used as a guide for management of the airway.
- Alternatives to direct laryngoscopy should be considered and used as back plans for anticipated difficult intubations.

- Considering the location of the vascular lesion and the level of obstruction can aid in determining the airway plan for intubating a patient for a procedure.
- Edema and hemorrhage are common complications associated with treatment of head and neck vascular lesions and should be accounted for when planning for extubation.

REFERENCES

1. White D, Harris G. Vascular neoplasms and malformations involving the airway. Facial Plast Surg 2012;28(06):590–5.

2. Rosenberg TL, Phillips JD. Update on vascular anomalies of the head and Neck. Otolaryngol Clin 2022;55(6):1215–31.

3. Klosterman T, Teresa MO. The management of vascular malformations of the airway. Otolaryngol Clin 2018;51(1):213–23.

4. Giese RA, Valero C, Shah JP. Surgical management of vascular tumors and malformations of the head and neck in adults. J Oral Pathol Med 2022;51(10):854–9.

5. Alsuwailem A, Myer CM, Chaudry G. Vascular anomalies of the head and Neck. Semin Pediatr Surg 2020;29(5):150968.

6. Castrén E, Aronniemi J, Klockars T, et al. Complications of sclerotherapy for 75 head and neck venous malformations. Eur Arch Oto-Rhino-Laryngol 2015;273(4):1027–36.

7. Jacobs IN, Cahill AM. Special considerations in vascular anomalies: Airway management. Clin Plast Surg 2011;38(1):121–31.

8. Clarke C, Lee E, Edmonds J. Vascular anomalies and airway concerns. Semin Plast Surg 2014;28(02):104–10.

9. Colletti G, Ierardi AM. Understanding venous malformations of the head and neck: A comprehensive insight. Med Oncol 2017;34(3):42.

10. Johnson AB, Richter GT. Surgical considerations in vascular malformations. Tech Vasc Intervent Radiol 2019;22(4):100635.

11. Bertino F, Trofimova AV, Gilyard SN, et al. Vascular anomalies of the head and neck: Diagnosis and treatment. Pediatr Radiol 2021;51(7):1162–84.

12. O'Dell K. Predictors of difficult intubation and the otolaryngology perioperative consult. Anesthesiol Clin 2015;33(2):279–90.

13. Apfelbaum JL, Hagberg CA, Connis RT, et al. 2022 American Society of Anesthesiologists Practice Guidelines for management of the difficult airway. Anesthesiology 2021;136(1):31–81.

14. Cooper RM. Strengths and limitations of airway techniques. Anesthesiol Clin 2015;33(2):241–55.

15. Law JA, Broemling N, Cooper RM, et al. The difficult airway with recommendations for management – part 2 – the anticipated difficult airway. Canadian Journal of Anesthesia/Journal canadien d'anesthésie 2013;60(11):1119–38.

16. Choi AM, Brenner MJ, Gorelik D, et al. New Medical Device and therapeutic approvals in otolaryngology: State of the Art Review of 2021. OTO Open 2022;6(3). 2473974X221126495.

Case Reviews in Head and Neck Vascular Lesion Management

Balasubramanya Kumar, MDS, FIBCSOMS[a],
Srinivasa R. Chandra, BDS, MD, FDS, FIBCSOMS(Onc-Recon)[b],*,
Sanjiv Nair, MDS, FDS, FFD[a],
Anjan Kumar Shah, MDS, FDS, FFD, FIBCSOMS(Onco & Recon)[a,c]

KEYWORDS

- Vascular lesions • Venous malformation • Cavernous hemangioma • Vascular malformation
- Bleomycin • Propranolol • Sirolimus • Beta-blocker

KEY POINTS

- Most vascular relations at some stage require surgical intervention status post-medical or interventional radiological therapy.
- Surgery has its challenges considering the location and access to most head and neck lesions.
- "Nidus" management by complete excision is the key to a high vascular lesion. The terminal feeders need to be occluded with litigation or deposition of any embolic material.
- Most of the tongue lesions present as low-flow lesions of a veno-lymphatic type and are rarely high-flow.
- Pericapsular dissection of a low-flow lesion is planned well with intralesional thrombotic agent injections and other interventional radiological techniques.

INTRODUCTION

This is a series of 6 cases representing the different management approaches to vascular lesions. The head and neck surgical subsites have been well represented with low flow and high flow and some distinct case theories that contribute to the presentation of the vascular lesion workup, approaches, and outcomes.[1-14]

Case 1

Low-flow vascular malformation of tongue

Presentation A 59-year-old man presented with an enormous swelling of the tongue for 25 years. The swelling had started causing difficulty in swallowing and speech. He reported occasional episodes of bleeding which were controlled with local measures (**Fig. 1**A–D).

Investigation MRI confirmed isolated involvement of tongue to determine the posterior extent of the lesion with little extension. Doppler and MRI confirmed low-flow vascular lesion.

Treatment The patient underwent anterior glossectomy with wide excision after collapsing the lesion with bilateral Satinsky vascular clamps applied on the tongue (see **Fig. 1**B) to compress the lesion thus aiding in limiting blood loss during surgery. Local oversewing and debulking of the lesion were carried out with monopolar cautery and usage of atraumatic resorbable sutures. He was on nasogastric feeds until swallowing, and

 a Maxillofacial Surgery, Bhagwan Mahaveer Jain Hospital, Bangalore, Karnataka, India; b Department of Maxillofacial-Head & Neck Oncologic and Reconstructive Microvascular Surgery, Oregon Health and Science University, Portland, OR, USA; c Oral & Maxillofacial Surgery, Rajarajeswari Dental College & Hospital, Bangalore, Karnataka, India
* Corresponding author. 3181 Southwest Sam Jackson Park Road, Portland, OR 97239.
E-mail address: chandrsr@ohsu.edu

Oral Maxillofacial Surg Clin N Am 36 (2024) 81–92
https://doi.org/10.1016/j.coms.2023.09.003
1042-3699/24/© 2023 Elsevier Inc. All rights reserved.

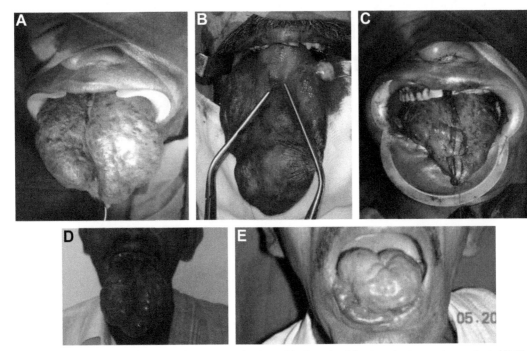

Fig. 1. Vascular control with 2 Satinsky clamps: This is an ideal method for transient vascular control. (*A*) Staged debulking of tongue with diffuse lesion discoloration. (*B*) Application of Satinsky clamps for vascular control and expeditious debulking. (*C*) Immediate postoperative appearance. Fig. 1D and E as described in patient case 1. (*D*) Preoperative illustration of rather large tongue lesion. (*E*) Postdebulking structural appearance of the tongue.

speech therapy was given. He was discharged and routine follow-up showed considerable improvement in his swallowing and speech.

This case illustrates how a lesion involving an isolated unit such as the tongue or lip can be managed with corseting and excision (**Fig. 1**A–E).

Learning points

- According to the authors' (Nair and colleagues) classification,[2,3] the aforementioned patient has a type I mucosal lesion.
- They are easy to diagnose as they frequently present with a bluish discoloration commonly seen with diffuse swelling.
- Most of these lesions can be completely excised in toto.
- Well-circumscribed tongue lesions are removed completely or debulked while trying to preserve the form and function of the tongue.
- Access through a V-shaped incision with the help of C or angled clamps not only helps in hemostasis but also enables primary closure.[14,15]

Case 2

Low-flow vascular malformation of the cheek
Presentation A 7-year-old child presented with swelling over the left side of his face. The swelling was soft, compressible, and non-pulsatile as a solitary mass (**Fig. 2**).

Investigation One of the few lesions where computed tomography (CT) could be helpful for diagnosis, a CT angiogram suggested a low-flow lesion involving the subcutaneous tissue overlying the left parotid and angle of the mandible (see **Fig. 2**B, C). The presence of phleboliths and details of feeding arteries were reviewed; nidus and draining veins were ruled out.

Treatment Considering the risk of damage to the facial nerve, it was decided to attempt conservative management with bleomycin. Ultrasound-guided injection was done to confirm the intralesional deposition of the drug. A 3-way syringe with a low caliber hypodermic needle is introduced into the lesion under ultrasound guidance. An amount of blood equal to the amount of drug to be administered is aspirated, and the precalculated dose of bleomycin is administered intralesionally.

2 such injections were performed with a gap interval of 3 months into the lesion (see **Fig. 2**E).

In 6 months, the lesion was almost completely resolved.

A 5-year follow-up has shown no recurrence (see **Fig. 2**D).

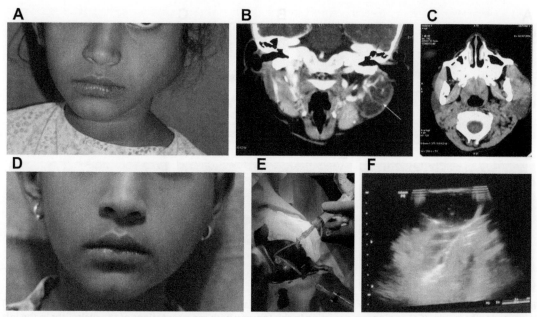

Fig. 2. Case 2: Low-flow malformation treated with ultrasound-guided intralesional bleomycin. (*A*) Left lower lateral facial mass with asymmetry. (*B*) Contrast enhanced computed tomography (CT) coronal section with the arrow depicting a left cystic parotid area lesion. (*C*) Contrast enhanced CT axial section with a left parotid lesion with mixed density after intralesional injections. (*D*) Left lower lateral facial mass resolved post therapy as noted in case 2 and injections demonstrated in Fig. 2E and F. (*E*) Intralesional injection with due aspiration and direct injection. (*F*) Ultrasound-guided injection of bleomycin.

In this case where the lesion is small, intralesional bleomycin using ultrasound was used for minimal morbidity and scarring.

Learning points
- Venous malformation usually presents as a symptomatic soft tissue mass.
- Though ultrasound is a useful tool in treating these lesions, a combination of ultrasound and CT angiography makes the dynamics of vascular malformations clearer.
- Bleomycin inhibits DNA synthesis and has a nonspecific inflammatory reaction on the endothelial cells.
- Though known to cause pulmonary fibrosis, the overall response is favorable.
- Intralesional injection of 15 IU bleomycin in 5 mL of fresh normal saline administered every 15 days for 3 to 4 sittings shows good result.[10,12,15]

Case 3

Low-flow vascular malformation of the face
Presentation A 50-year-old man presented with a diffuse swelling over the right side of his face, progressively getting larger and more painful (**Fig. 3**A).

Investigation A CT angiogram showed a low-flow lesion with multiple vascular channels involving the cheek, masseter, and parotid gland along with multiple phleboliths (**Fig. 3**B).

The presence of phleboliths within a soft tissue mass on CT is a characteristic of venous malformation. The serpiginous enhancement involving multiple compartments is suggestive of low-flow vascular malformation.[14,15]

Treatment A preauricular incision with a cervical extension was used to access the lesion. Wide excision and corseting to strangulate the deeper part of the lesion was done to reduce the bulk of the lesion. Placement of a bioresorbable suture (polydioxanone) in a continuous vertical looping fashion constricts the tumor thus obliterating the blood circulation. The excess skin was then excised to achieve closure (**Fig. 3**C–F).

Outcome The lesion reduced in size considerably in 3 months.

There was transient facial palsy which resolved in 6 months.

Learning points
- Low-flow lesions involving more diffuse areas where complete excision is not possible can be managed with a combination of excision and corseting sutures to reduce morbidity.

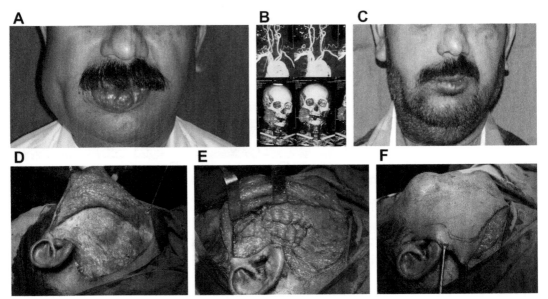

Fig. 3. (*A, B*) Low-flow venous vascular malformation of the face. (*A*) Right lateral masseteric area facial mass. (*B*) Computed tomography (CT) angiogram depicting in the top row with representations of the pleboliths in the left facial region noted as white satellite clusters; Images at the bottom row of the CT angiogram depict the large venous malformation with circuitous channels and pleboliths. (*C*) Postsurgical intervention with staged corsetting and resection of the lesion. Please note transient right facial weakness. (*D*) Case 3: a preauricular incision with flap elevation for a low-flow venous vascular malformation of the face. (*E*) Case 3: low-flow venous vascular malformation of the face, with placement of 'corset sutures' to obliterate the lesion. (*F*) Case 3: low-flow venous vascular malformation of the face with removal of excess skin status post resection of expansile venous malformation in the right parotid area.

- Corset suturing is a proven technique, especially where important structures like the facial nerve are involved.[3,14]
- Large lesions require further excision and debulking as age advances and lesions linger.
- Large low-flow lesions have a potential to be completely removed at a second stage once shrinkage is achieved by corseting.
- Noncapsulated lesions are then rarely excised completely but improve the quality of life and reduce the risk of mortality due to pressure symptoms on the airway and hemorrhage.

Case 4

High-flow lesion of lip

Presentation A 60-year-old man presented with a pulsatile swelling of the lower lip with occasional bleeding for which he had to get emergency surgical treatment (**Fig. 4**).

On examination, there was a soft, compressible swelling involving the lower lip, left commissure, and chin region. There was a palpable bruit.

A handheld Doppler ultrasound confirmed high-flow lesion of the face.

Investigation CT angiogram showed isolated feeder vessels coming from the left facial artery.

Compression of the facial artery at the mandible angle reduced the Doppler signal in the lesion (see **Fig. 4**B).

An MRI also confirmed the anatomic extent of the lesion. It was infiltrating the subcutaneous tissues but showed to extension into the underlying bone.

Treatment The common carotid and external carotid artery (ECA) were identified, and the branches of the ECA were dissected but preserved. A vascular clamp (No 1 bulldog) was placed on the facial artery trunk, and simultaneously Doppler signal in the lip lesion was evaluated. There was a reduction in signal intensity of the Doppler, confirming arterial supply mainly from the facial artery. Wide excision of the lesion under carotid artery control was done.

The remaining lip commissure was recreated using the redundant lip tissue and rotation to close. The excess skin was closed using a rotation advancement flap of the neck skin (see **Fig. 4**I).

Outcome Lesion healed uneventfully. In 6 months, the commissure function was almost back to normal with very little drooling of saliva following treatment.

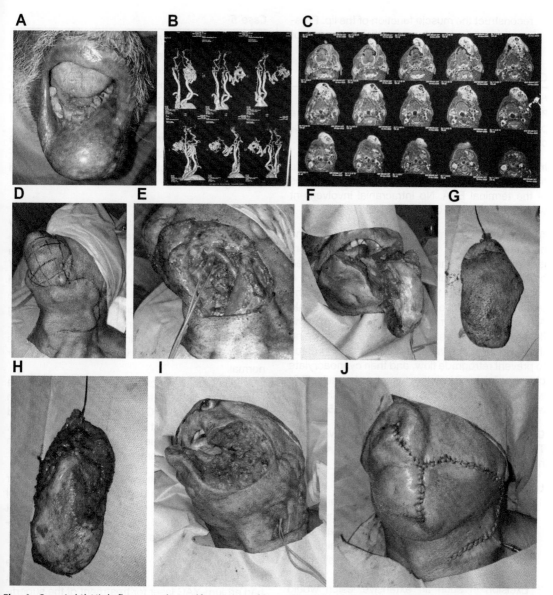

Fig. 4. Case 4: (*A*) High-flow vascular malformation of lower lip with asymmetry. Fig. 4B of case 4: Preoperative CT angiogram showing isolated feeders from ECA. Fig. 4C of Case 4: Preoperative contrasted MRI scan axial views demonstrating the intense vascular perfusion, flow voids, and lip deformation. Fig. 4D of Case 4: planned surgical incision and area of the lesion cross hatched for excision; (*E*) High-flow vascular malformation of lower lip with asymmetry. External carotid artery identification and control with vascular loop. (*F–H*) High-flow vascular malformation of lower lip excision. (*F*) Intraoperative picture with ECA control and post excision; (*G, H*) cutaneous and mucosal surface. Case 4: (*I*) High-flow vascular malformation of lower lip excision defect; (*J*) Neck and lower lip immediate closure post excision.

No recurrence of the lesion has been seen on follow-up of 2 years (see **Fig. 4**).

Learning points

1. This case illustrates in a high-flow lesion, if the vascular territory shows isolated feeders, how vascular ECA control and excision can be done to treat such lesions.
2. It is important to note that this type of treatment is possible when a well demarcated, isolated

high-flow lesion is identified. MRI is the most useful tool for determining the extent of the lesion.

3. Complete excision of the 'nidus' or vascular shunted tissue gives the best chance of cure. In the head and neck region this is difficult as several vital structures are present, and excision can cause significant deformity.
4. A local flap as illustrated provides the best result for lip function, as no distant flap can

reconstruct the muscle function of the lip. Preservation of lip function was the main goal of reconstruction in this case.

Case 5

High-flow lesion scalp
Presentation A 45-year-old lady presented with a pulsatile swelling of her right scalp. The lesion occasionally bled while combing her hair (**Fig. 5**A).

Investigation A CT angiogram showed multiple high-flow channels in the scalp fed by branches of the terminal ECA. No intracranial involvement was noted (**Fig. 5**B, C).

Treatment Using direct vascular access from the neck, the ECA was exposed. The carotid artery is first identified, and then the ECA is identified by the presence of branches in the neck. A vascular clamp (No 1 bulldog) was placed on the terminal ECA, above the facial and lingual trunk. A handheld Doppler is used to confirm that the flow signal in the lesion shuts down on clamping these vessels. The vascular clamp is left in place to prevent retrograde flow, and then cyanoacrylate glue was injected into the vascular channels. This was allowed to set, and then the lesion was excised, and corset sutures placed (**Fig. 5**D–M).

Outcome The surgical site healed uneventfully. The patient followed up for 1 year and showed no recurrence of the lesion.

Learning points
1. As the lesion was overlying the cranium, a CT angiogram was the most appropriate investigation to rule out intracranial communications of the lesion. The CT angiogram also helps map out the vascular tree of the lesion, assisting in the approach to access the vessels.
2. Excision of such an extensive lesion would have resulted in a very large defect which would require microvascular free tissue transfer. It was therefore decided to use a more conservative approach. Transfemoral catheterization and embolization of terminal branches is a technically challenging procedure, and possible retrograde flow risks the embolic glue to enter the internal carotid artery with disastrous consequences, such as stroke.
3. This case illustrates how in a high-flow lesion, which is more extensive and where embolization would involve multiple catheterizations, local embolization with glue into the lesion itself may shut down feeders before excision.
4. The cyanoacrylate glue if left in the tissues can sometimes cause a foreign body reaction and necessitate further excision.

Case 6

High-flow lesions: lip and chin subunits
Presentation A 26-year-old patient presented with a swelling of the lower lip and chin with skin color changes (**Fig. 6**). There was a marked bruit over the chin. Previous ligation of the facial artery had not significantly reduced size of lesion (see **Fig. 6**A).

Investigation CT angiogram showed multiple feeders from branches of the ECA. No intraosseous extension of the vascular channels noted (see **Fig. 6**B).

Treatment
Surgery 1 The ECA was exposed to identify feeding vessels. It was noted that a large 'facial artery like' vessel had developed since previous facial artery ligation. A vascular clamp (No 1 bulldog) was applied to the vessel, and reduced signal intensity was noted in the facial lesion. The bulk of the lesion was excised, and the remaining part of the lesion was strangulated with corseting.

A significant reduction in size of the lesion was noted and lip function was returned to near normal.

A follow-up 3 years later however, showed a recurrence of a pulsatile lesion in the chin area in cutaneous regions. A CT angiogram scan revealed that the lip component of the lesion had regressed, but a large high-flow lesion in the skin of the chin persisted. No intra-bony extension was noted.

Surgery 2 Embolization of multiple vascular feeding channels was done with polyvinyl alcohol particles. 2 days post embolization, the patient had wide excision of the subcutaneous component of the lesion (see **Fig. 6**D).

Outcome Significant reduction in the size of the lesion was observed in 3 months. The patient had erbium-YAG laser for treatment of the superficial lesions of the skin.

Learning points
1. The treatment for a high-flow lesion in the head and neck region is not ligation of the facial artery. Ligations prevent the possibility of insertion of a catheter for embolization if necessary in the future.
2. Excision of the 'nidus' is the treatment of choice for high-flow vascular malformation.
3. Allowing the arterial branches to remain patent after excision of the lesions provides embolization access if required for these patients.
4. This case illustrates how for large, diffuse high-flow lesions, combined approach with embolization and excision can be used to reduce morbidity.

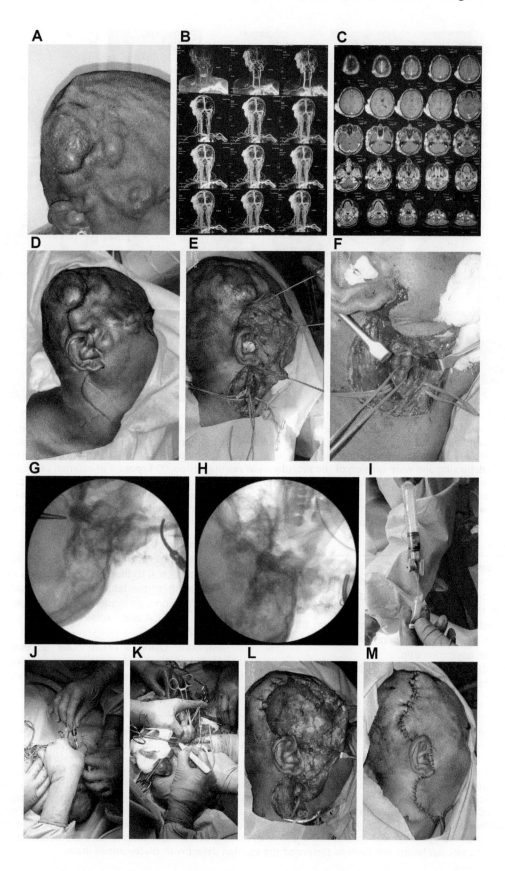

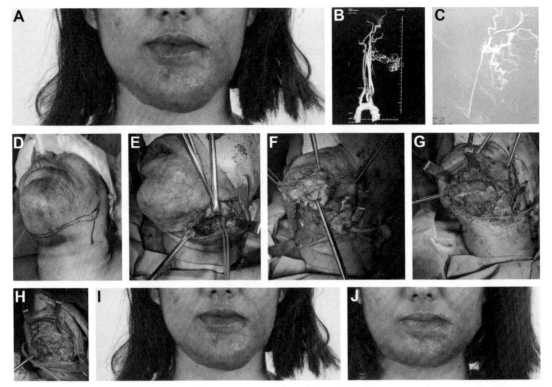

Fig. 6. Case 6: (*A*) High-flow vascular malformation involving chin and lip. (*B*) computed tomography (CT) angiogram showed multiple feeders from branches of the external carotid artery (ECA). No intra-osseous extension of the vascular channels noted. (*C*) Embolization of multiple vascular feeding channels was done with polyvinyl alcohol (PVA) particles. (*D*) Surgical incision marking 2 days post embolization. (*E*) Exposure of carotid control prior to debulking and wide excision of the subcutaneous vascular lesion. (*F*) Exposure of external carotid artery and control prior to debulking and wide excision of the subcutaneous vascular lesion. (*G*) Excision and corseting of residual lesion. (*H*) Completion of excision and debulking of the vascular lesion. Case 6: (*I*) Preoperative lip and chin area vascular lesion. (*J*) Postsurgical excision of the facial subunit regions with ongoing laser therapy for pigment reduction caused by vascular lesion of the subcutaneous areas.

Case 7

Arteriovenous malformation

Presentation A 37-year-old male presented with 4 × 4 cm compressible, pulsatile swelling in left cheek for 10 years duration, warm to palpate with distinct bruit. No discolorations on the skin over the swelling were obvious. Otherwise, the patient was asymptomatic.

Investigation: US Doppler identified the high-flow arterial supply into the lesion with cavernous sac. Magnetic resonance anigiography and digital subtraction angiography demonstrated a sizable venous sac lateral to the pterygo-maxillary region with feeders from the facial and internal maxillary (**Fig. 7**). Decision was made to gain intraoperative control on the ECA and excise the venous sac[9–14] (see **Fig. 7**B).

Treatment: Using a preauricular access with cervical and temporal extension the facial flap was raised at the superficial musculoaponeurotic

Fig. 5. (*A*) High-flow vascular malformation of right scalp, with scarring from prior ulcerations and bleeds. (*B*) With a collage of the computed tomography angiogram (CTA) with vascular lesions in the tempero-parietal area. (*C*) CTA showing no intracranial feeders noted on the axial section of the CTA. (*D*) Right scalp lesion surgical marking of planned incision and excision areas; (*E*) External carotid artery (ECA) isolated and feeder vessels injected with cyanoacrylate glue for embolization and placement of corset sutures in the right parotid bed area; (*F*) Intraoperative external carotid control with vessel loops. Case 5: (*G, H*) Intraoperative fluoroscopic images utilizing a C arm reviewing the embolization after ECA access. Case 5: (*I*) Cyanoacrylate glue obtained into a syringe with flow valve, (*J*) Accessing the vascular lesion for injection of cyanoacrylate to 'dam' the outflow; (*K*) excision of the scalp lesion post vascular control and injection of tissue glue; (*L*) Right scalp to neck exposure with resection of the vascular lesion; (*M*) Esthetic closure of the excision defect with placement of drain.

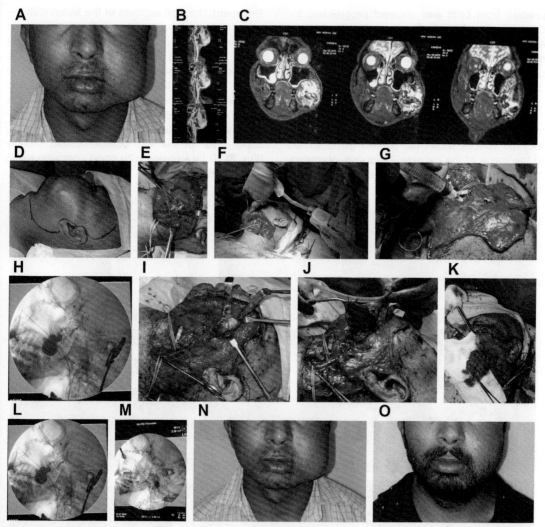

Fig. 7. Case 7: (*A–C*) Clockwise. (*A*) Arteriovenous malformation (AVM) of the left cheek. (*B*) Magnetic resonance angiography (MRA) and digital subtractiob angiography (DSA) demonstrated the size of the venous sac lateral to the pterygo-maxillary region with feeders from the facial and internal maxillary. (*C*) Coronal section of the MRA with large multiloculated sac of the vascular AVM. Case 7: (*D*) Extended planned incision into the neck for external carotid artery (ECA) access. (*E*) Intraoperative control the ECA and excise the venous sac. Case 7: (*F*) Intraoperative Doppler to identify changes in flow with ECA control and gradual embolization techniques. (*G*) Intraoperative ECA control and gradual embolization technique. (*H*) Vascular AVM embolized as demonstrated with the intraoperative fluoroscopic C arm technique. (*I*) ECA control, intermittent bull dog clamping, and dissection with identification of facial nerve branches allowed complete access. (*J, K*) Demonstration and excision of the large vascular AVM sac after ligating the vascular pedicle was done. (*L*) Preoperative AVM sac: (pointed by the *thick blue arrow* after cyanoacrylate injection). (*M*) Post excision of the sac (pointed by the *thick blue arrow* after cyanoacrylate injection). (*N*) Preoperative facial photograph of the left facial mass. (*O*) Postoperative facial picture of the area with residual edema.

system layer. The ECA was identified and controlled with vascular clamps. Intraoperatively contrast was injected into the feeders to identify the venous sac using a C arm image (see **Fig. 7**G, H). Cyanoacrylate glue was injected into the sac to solidify the lesion. Blunt dissection with identification of facial nerve branches allowed complete excision after ligating the vascular

pedicle was done. Good cosmetic and functional result was achieved.

Case 8

Lymphatic malformation or lymphovenous malformation
Presentation Female, 25 years of age, with swelling in the preauricular region, which was

present from birth and showed progressive increase in size. The swelling had the shape of an enlarged parotid gland clinically indicating its presence within the capsule of the parotid gland. It was previously operated during childhood with unsuccessful attempt at removal.

Investigation CT angiograph demonstrated macrocystic spaces within the parotid gland limited to the inside of the capsule. Diagnosis of macrocystic lymphatic malformation was arrived at.

Treatment Surgical excision of the lesion with the superficial parotid was planned. Through a parotid incision a facial flap along the parotid fascia was raised. The gland with its enclosed lesion was exposed. Facial nerve was identified tracing the upper border of the posterior belly of digastric muscle. The lesion could be peeled off of the branches of the facial nerve with ease. The preauricular soft tissue defect was filled by swinging the upper layer of the sternocleidomastoid muscle (**Fig. 8**). Total excision with good cosmetic result was achieved.[3,9,13]

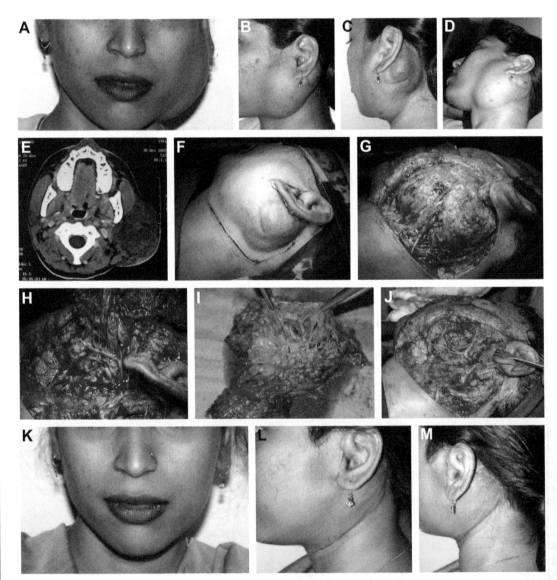

Fig. 8. (*A–D*) Left facial vascular lesion of *lymphatic malformation or lymphovenous malformation type*. (*E*) CT scan of the axial image depicting the large multicystic lesion (macrocystic spaces within the parotid gland). (*F–J*) (*Left top*: Clockwise). (*F*) Intraoperative pictures of incision; (*G*) flap elevation; (*H*) identification of the facial nerve; (*I*) cystic sac of the mass with multilocation excision; (*J*) Postexcision left parotid bed with adequate hemostasis; Case 8: (*K–M*) Postoperative frontal, lateral, and left posterior facial area and neck incision areas.

Learning points

1. Arteriovenous malformations (AVMs) are treated as 2 separate entities; hence, controlling the arterial flow and excision of the venous sac gives satisfactory outcome.
2. Use of ECA control over transosseous-alveolar embolization can prove to be effective in AVMs especially considering that a lot of embolic particles may disappear into the venous system.
3. Preauricular or buccal lesions need careful identification and isolation of facial nerve branches.
4. Incisions to the lesion require meticulous planning for complete access and ablation of the lesion.
5. Glandular lesions would require excision with the gland rather than dissecting the vascular lesion from within the parenchyma of the gland.

SUMMARY

Vascular lesions of the head and neck are reviewed for surgical excision and management based on our departmental publications and protocols led by Nair and colleagues.[3,4,9,13] This classification of 5 types is based on the location from skin subcutaneous tissue, muscular or subcutaneous, glandular, intra-osseous, and deep visceral areas of anatomy. This simple anatomic and surgical classification proposes a management as represented in the cases earlier.

CLINICS CARE POINTS

- In high-flow lesions, where more extensive need embolization, multiple catheterizations, local embolization with glue direct into the lesion may shut down small feeders before excision.

- The treatment for a high-flow lesion in the head and neck region is not ligation of the facial artery or similar major branches. Ligations prevent the possibility of insertion of a catheter for embolization if necessary in the future.

- Arteriovenous malformations (AVMs) are treated as 2 separate entities; hence, controlling the arterial flow and excision of the venous sac gives satisfactory outcome.

- Glandular lesions would require excision with the gland rather than dissecting the vascular lesion from within the parenchyma of the gland.

- Cyanoacrylate glue if left in the tissues can sometimes cause a foreign body reaction and necessitate further excision.

DISCLOSURE

No disclosures are reported for any of the authors.

REFERENCES

1. Mulliken JB, Fishman SJ, Burrows PE. Vascular anomalies. Curr Probl Surg 2000;37:517.
2. Saint-Jean M, Léauté-Labrèze C, Mazereeuw-Hautier J, et al. Propranolol for treatment of ulcerated infantile hemangiomas. J Am Acad Dermatol 2011;64:827.
3. Nair SC, Chandra SR. Management of head and neck vascular lesions: a guide for surgeons. 1st edition. Springer Nature; 2022. https://doi.org/10.1007/978-981-15-2321-2.
4. Nair SC. Vascular Anomalies of the Head and Neck Region. J Maxillofac Oral Surg 2018;17:1–12.
5. Waner M, Suen JY. Hemangiomas and vascular malformations of the head and neck. Wiley-Liss; 1999.
6. Mulliken JB, Glowacki J. Hemangiomas and vascular malformations in infants and children: a classification based on endothelial characteristics. P Reconstr Surg 1982;69(3):412–22.
7. Ethunandan M, Mellor TK. Hemangiomas and vascular malformations of the maxillofacial region – review. Br J Maxillofac Surg 2006;44:263–72.
8. Venot Q, Blanc T, Rabia SH, et al. Targeted therapy in patients with PIK3CA-related overgrowth syndrome. Nature 2018;558(7711):540–6.
9. Chandra SR, Nair S. History, terminology, and classifications of vascular anomalies-pages 1-9, management of head and neck vascular lesions: a guide for surgeons. 1st edition. Springer Nature; 2022. https://doi.org/10.1007/978-981-15-2321-2.
10. Chandra SR, Kumar B, Shroff S, et al. Pathogenesis, genetics, and molecular developments in vascular lesion therapy and diagnosis, pages 11-27; management of head and neck vascular lesions: a guide for surgeons. 1st edition. Springer Nature; 2022. https://doi.org/10.1007/978-981-15-2321-2.
11. Chandra SR, Yu L, Ghodke B. Radiological diagnosis of head and neck vascular anomalies, pages 49-65, management of head and neck vascular lesions: a guide for surgeons. 1st edition. Springer Nature; 2022. https://doi.org/10.1007/978-981-15-2321-2.
12. Chandra SR, Kumar J, Nair SC. Medical management of vascular lesions: current and the future, pages 67-103, management of head and neck vascular lesions: a guide for surgeons. 1st edition. Springer Nature; 2022. https://doi.org/10.1007/978-981-15-2321-2.
13. Chandra SR, Shroff S, Curry S, et al. General, surgical, and functional anatomy for vascular lesions of

head and neck, pages 105-135; management of head and neck vascular lesions: a guide for surgeons. 1st edition. Springer Nature; 2022. https://doi.org/10.1007/978-981-15-2321-2.

14. Nair SC, Shroff S, Chandra SR. Surgical management, pages 137-157, management of head and neck vascular lesions: a guide for surgeons. 1st

edition. Springer Nature; 2022. https://doi.org/10.1007/978-981-15-2321-2.

15. Burt J, Rodriguez-Vasquez J, Ghodke B, et al. The role of interventional radiology, pages 67-103; management of head and neck vascular lesions: a guide for surgeons. 1st edition. Springer Nature; 2022. https://doi.org/10.1007/978-981-15-2321-2.

Updates to the Management of Gorham–Stout Disease and Osseous Vascular Lesions in the Head and Neck

Andrea B. Burke, DMD, MD[a],*, Chao Dong, MS[b],
Srinivasa R. Chandra, BDS, MD, FDSRCS, FIBCSOMS (Oncology-Recons)[c]

KEYWORDS

- Vascular tumor • Hemangioma • Disappearing bone • Lymphangiomatosis
- Gorham–Stout disease • Intraosseous hemangioma • Epithelioid hemangioma
- Pseudomyogenic hemangioendothelioma

KEY POINTS

- Osseous vascular tumors are rare and are classified based on their biological potential.
- Gorham-Stout disease is a rare disease marked by the disintegration of bone structure, the growth of lymphatic vascular formations, and extensive localized bone degradation.
- Treatment of vascular and lymphatic malformations involves the use of embolic agents, surgery, laser, and developing medical therapies.
- The PI3KCA/AKT/mTOR pathway may yield future therapeutic potential for vascular anomalies and Gorham–Stout disease.

OSSEOUS VASCULAR ANOMALIES

Osseous vascular tumors are categorized based on their biological potential: benign hemangiomas, epithelioid hemangiomas (intermediate-locally aggressive), pseudomyogenic hemangioendothelioma (intermediate-rarely metastasizing), malignant epithelioid hemangioendothelioma, and angiosarcoma (**Table 1**).[1] Vascular tumors arise from abnormalities in endothelial cell proliferation. The most common osseous vascular tumors of the cranium are benign hemangiomas, which commonly present as radiolucencies in the spine and long bones, with a prevalence of about 10%, and rarely leading to neurologic deficits. Conversely, infantile hemangiomas, which do not usually involve bone, typically seem early in infancy and undergo proliferation until

approximately 1 year of age when they begin to involute, a process that can take many years.

The role of the age is significant in that most benign osseous hemangiomas are asymptomatic and found in pediatric populations, whereas metastatic lesions are found more commonly in adults.[1,2] Primary vascular lesions of the jaws are rare in children, with most involving other tissues. Aneurysmal bone cysts and central vascular malformations (eg, Rendu–Osler–Weber syndrome) have been reported as primary vascular lesions of the jaws in the pediatric population.

PHACE(S) is a syndrome that includes posterior fossa malformation, hemangioma, arterial anomalies, coarctation of aorta and cardiac anomalies, and eye defects (and sternal raphe). Most (90%)

---

[a] Oral and Maxillofacial Surgery, University of Washington School of Dentistry, 1959 Northeast Pacific Street, Box 357134, Seattle, WA 98195-7134, USA; [b] University of Washington School of Dentistry; [c] Oral & Maxillofacial Surgery–Head Neck Oncology/Microvascular Reconstruction, Oregon Health & Science University
* Corresponding author.
E-mail address: abburke@uw.edu

Oral Maxillofacial Surg Clin N Am 36 (2024) 93–102
https://doi.org/10.1016/j.coms.2023.09.004
1042-3699/24/© 2023 Elsevier Inc. All rights reserved.

of the patients with this syndrome have more than one extracutaneous manifestation, with significant head and neck involvement. About 40% of these patients have infantile hemangiomas, and many become symptomatic. Importantly, the hemangiomas can be subglottic or involve the airway. MRI/MRA can be used to evaluate cerebral malformations.

It is important to determine whether a maxillofacial vascular abnormality is a tumor versus a malformation, as this can affect prognosis and treatment.[1,2] Malformations grow by expanding the bone and causing dilation. Most vascular lesions involving bone are malformations that will cause bony destruction or distortion. Vascular malformations are present at birth and will grow proportionately with the patient; however, intraosseous malformations typically do not become evident until later in life.

Vascular anomalies occur frequently in children; however, confusing nomenclature and a lack of pathophysiologic understanding has led to difficulty in diagnosis and treatment of these lesions.[3] Mulliken and Glowacki[4] proposed a biologic classification of vascular anomalies in 1982, separating vascular tumors from vascular malformations (slow vs fast flow).[5]

The radiographic features of all vascular tumors of bone are typically lytic and occasionally lytic-mixed sclerotic (**Fig. 1**). Hemangiomas can often be diagnosed by radiographic appearance alone, but angiosarcomas are aggressive and infiltrative in appearance. Histologic features are usually smooth borders, lobulation, and vasoformation in the benign subtypes, with more infiltrative and ragged appearance in the malignant subtypes, with the absence of lobulation or vasoformation. Epithelioid hemangiomas may be mistaken for common hemangiomas, but histology shows more than half of the tumors cells as epithelioid, as opposed to a majority of bland endothelial cells.

The Fos gene family, encoding for the transcription factor FOS (Fos Proto-Oncogene, AP-1 Transcription Factor Subunit) and its parlogue, FOSB, have been described in osseous vascular tumors, such as osteoblastoma and pseudomyogenic hemangioendothelioma. Epithelioid hemangiomas, on some occasions, share similar mutations. YAP1-TFE3 (Yes1 Associated Transcriptional Regulator - Transcription Factor Binding To IGHM Enhancer 3) and WWTR1-CAMTA1 (WW Domain Containing Transcription Regulator 1 - Calmodulin Binding Transcription Activator 1) genetic rearrangements are known to cause epithelioid hemangioma endotheliomas. Additionally, EWSR1-NFATC1 (EWS RNA Binding Protein 1 - Nuclear Factor Of Activated T Cells 1) fusion variations have been documented in hemangioma of the bone. Endothelial cells are used for immunohistochemical markers for occasional confirmation of skeletal lesions.[2]

The markers prox1 (Prospero Homeobox 1), podpplanin, ERG (ETS Transcription Factor ERG), FLI1 (Fli-1 Proto-Oncogene), surface antigens CD34 and CD31 are commonly used. Future work is being performed to look for bone-specific immunohistochemical markers.

Prognosis

Primary hemangioma of the bone is rare and often misrepresented. Venous intraosseous lesions are managed by "insightful neglect" if the lesion is not of a significant volume with no substantial clinical problems. Epithelioid hemangioma is commonly mistaken for hemangioma as more than half of the neoplastic cellular content is epithelioid unlike hemangiomas which contain bland endothelial cells and fewer epithelioid cells.

Angiosarcoma which is the other interosseous vascular tumor is an aggressive and infiltrative malignancy causing significant clinical symptoms and with a high suspicion adequate imaging and biopsy could confirm.

GORHAM–STOUT DISEASE

Gorham–Stout disease (GSD) is a sporadic bone disorder characterized by progressive bone resorption and possible malignant proliferation of vascular (lymphatic) structures. GSD is also known as disappearing bone disease, vanishing bone disease, and more than a dozen other terms in medical literature. As such, it is closely related to lymphangiomatosis.

In 1838, J B S Jackson, an American surgeon and pathologist, first reported the condition titled

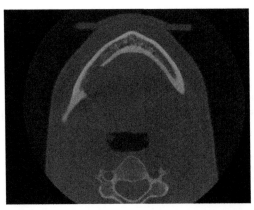

Fig. 1. The radiographic features of all vascular tumors of bone are typically lytic and occasionally lytic-mixed sclerotic.

"A Boneless Arm" in *The Boston Medical and Surgical Journal* (now The New England Journal of Medicine).[6–8] Although the humerus bone had diminished in size and shortened length, the patient reported using the arm well.[2] In 1954, Dr Gorham and Dr Stout hypothesized that angiomatosis was responsible for this unusual bone resorption after publishing two case series and reviewing 16 similar cases.[7–12] They presented the abstract to the American Association of Physicians in the same year. In October 1955, "Massive Osteolysis (Acute Spontaneous Absorption of Bone, Phantom Bone, Disappearing Bone): Its Relation to Hemangiomatosis" was published in *The Journal of Bone and Joint Surgery*. In a series of 24 patients, it was hypothesized that this disease is associated with angiomatosis of blood and sometimes of lymphatic vessels.

Genetics/Etiology/Epidemiology

The etiology and pathophysiology of GSD remains poorly understood, with no environmental or genetic risk factors having been identified. Gorham and Stout defined the disease as hemangiomatosis, which includes hyperemia and bone destruction. Heyden suggested that local hypoxia and acidosis caused increased activity of hydrolytic enzymes, and Young thought the osteolysis came from local endothelial dysplasia.[10,11] Recent hypotheses consider the enhanced osteoclastic activity secondary to increased IL-6, IL-1, and TNF.[11–15] IL-6 is capable of stimulating osteoclast activity and increasing sensitivity of osteoclast precursors to humoral factors, such as IL-1 and TNF.[14,15] The strong activity of both acid phosphatase and leucine aminopeptidase in mononuclear perivascular cells that are in contact with remaining bone, perhaps indicating these cells are important in the process of osseous resorption. Several reports also described an overlap between visceral and bone lymphangiomatosis.[12]

GSD occurs sporadically, with symptoms appearing at any age, any race, and any gender. Most cases have been reported under age 40 years, with children and young adults mostly affected. Symptoms vary depending on the bones affected and can range from mild to severe, even life-threatening.[12–15]

There is currently no standardization for diagnosing GSD. Currently, the diagnosis is made by histopathological and clinical correlation, with the following eight diagnostic criteria.

1. Positive histologic findings for proliferation and angiomatous dysplasia
2. Absence of osteoblastic reaction and/or dystrophic calcifications
3. Evidence of local bone progressive resorption

4. Exclusion of cellular atypia
5. Non-ulcerative lesion
6. Absence of visceral involvement
7. Osteolytic radiographic pattern
8. Negative hereditary, metabolic, neoplastic, immunologic, and infectious etiology

Clinical Presentation and Subtypes

GSD may affect multiple bones, but in most cases, it stays in one region of the body.[12,14] The most common symptoms are pain and swelling in the affected area, with no apparent cause. In some cases, pathologic fractures may be the first presenting symptom. Pathologic fractures may be characterized by sclerosis around the fracture site, and screening for post-fracture acceleration of bone resorption in these patients is important. Bones commonly affected by GSD include ribs, spine, pelvis, skull, clavicle, shoulder, and jaws.[14,15] Approximately 30% of affected patients had maxillofacial involvement, with mandible being the most frequently affected jawbone. The most common finding is pain and swelling on the affected area. Other findings include mobile teeth, malocclusion, deviation of mandible, facial deformity, and occasional pathologic fractures. Laboratory studies can be completely within normal limits. Patients with spine and skull involvement may experience neurologic complications, acute spinal pain, and paralysis, with occasional spinal fluid leakage. If the ribs or thoracic vertebrae are involved, the known findings include breathing difficulty, chest pain, weight loss, and chylothorax.

Radiographic Findings

The radiologic appearance of bone lesions reveals intramedullary and subcortical radiolucency. The classic radiologic features of GDS are tapering bone ends or a "mouse tail" appearance. GSD can be categorized into four distinct radiographic stages: The first stage shows patchy osteopenia in the intramedullary or subcortical regions resembling osteoporosis. At the second stage, confluent radiolucencies produce new broader radiolucent areas.[16] The third stage is characterized by the involvement of adjacent soft tissue after cortical breakage. At the final stage, the involved bone is completely resorbed and replaced by fibrous tissue (**Fig. 2**).

Computed tomography is useful to evaluate bony destruction, and MRI can distinctly depict the extent of lesion, with a heterogeneous peripheral gadolinium enhancement. Differential diagnosis from imaging includes malignant tumors, such as Ewing's sarcoma, metastasis, osteosarcoma, or multiple myeloma. Bone scintigraphy and whole-body PET

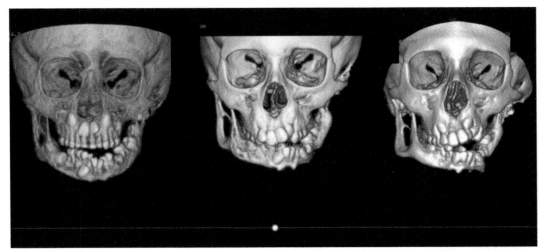

Fig. 2. Destruction of normal cortical architecture of the mandibular condyle, ramus, and body more than 6 years.

imaging can reflect the bone metabolic activity of a regional lesion and are useful in ruling out neoplastic or infective pathology. Recently, fluorine-18-sodium fluoride PET/CT has been proposed as a more bone-specific agent than fluorine-18-fluoro-D-glucose PET/CT, particularly in the assessment of disease activity and treatment response.[17,18]

Histologic Findings

The first histologic stage is vascular proliferation, and the second involves fibrous tissue replacing resorbed bone. In early stages, tissue removed from radiolucent defects consists of a nonspecific vascular proliferation intermixed with fibrous connective tissue and a chronic inflammatory cell infiltrate composed of lymphocytes and plasma cells. Vascular proliferation is characterized by thin-walled channels. Osteoclastic reaction in adjacent bone fragments is usually not noted (**Fig. 3**). Based on the idea that GSD is the bone version of lymphangiomatosis, staining for lymphatic vessel endothelial hyaluronan receptor-1 and CD31 is often done to aid in diagnosis.

TREATMENT STRATEGIES

Treatment of maxillofacial vascular anomalies depends on their type (tumor or malformation), clinical staging, location, and symptoms. Critical anatomic location, signs of infection, fluid leakage, thrombosis, fluctuation in size, bleeding, and so forth should be considered. Some malformations can lead to pain and functional impairment, inhibiting quality of life.

Many infantile hemangiomas can be treated with observation as they involute, though sometimes local treatment is required for ulceration or bleeding. Corticosteroids, local injection for smaller lesions and systemic administration for larger lesions, interferon alpha-2a or 2b, or vincristine have been used for treatment.[1,7,11] Surgery may be indicated for well-localized tumors, but treatment may also be staged.[13]

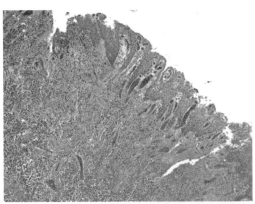

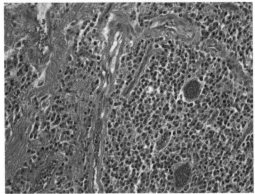

Fig. 3. GSD histology: vascular proliferation of thin-walled endothelial capillaries within bone. Extreme thinning of bony trabeculae. Resorption and replacement of bone with angiomas and/or fibrosis.

Management of vascular malformations depends on whether lesions are slow flow or fast flow. Capillary malformations, such as those seen in Sturge–Weber syndrome, can be monitored. The concomitant bony overgrowth that can occur may need to be treated with recontouring or orthodontia. Venous malformations, which are the most common anomaly in the jaws, can be treated with combined orthodontics/orthognathic surgery in mild cases. Consumptive coagulopathy, due to stasis and turbulence of vasculature, can be treated with heparin or antifibrinolytic agents. Larger lesions benefit from sclerosing agents, discussed below.

Arteriovenous malformations, which are fast flow, may be associated with loose teeth or bleeding. They can undergo acute changes in size and compress critical anatomic structures. Ultrasound with Doppler and MRI/MRA/MRV can be useful to determine the extent of the lesion.[16–18] Embolization of lesions has changed the management of these lesions, with arterial embolization followed by surgical resection, to help combat their high recurrence rates.

Interventional Radiology

Interventional radiology can be used in both the identification and treatment of osseous proliferative vascular anomalies. Once the immunochemistry has been confirmed to be a nonmalignant lesion based on the list mentioned above in diagnosis, then they can be treated as listed below. Minimally invasive techniques have helped to reduce morbidity in many cases.

Embolization is based on the concept of rheology and the physics of slow flow versus rapid. If a lesion is slow flow at the area of direct puncture, sclerosing liquid agents and additional medical treatments can be performed. The subsequent venous outflow control is obtained using a venting technique.[19] High-flow arteriovenous malformations are considered for embolization if the nidus can be accessed. If the embolization alone is inadequate, surgery must also be considered for complete resection.

Ethanol with a direct puncture can be performed for venous, venolymphatic, and small localized arteriovenous malformations.[20] Ethanol is an irritant, and extreme care is advised. Endovascular access may be necessary in some lesions. Polidocanol (Aetoxisclerol) is a sclerosing agent that was first developed as a local anesthetic and causes vascular spasm. Bleomycin can be used as an intralesional injection, directly into malformations, but carries the risk of pulmonary toxicity with cumulative dosing. Onyx (ethylene vinyl alcohol) is a nonadhesive and cohesive liquid embolic agent dissolved in dimethyl sulfoxide.[19,21] It is nonresorbable polymer that gradually solidifies within the vessel to form an intravascular plug. It does not stick to the vessel walls, permitting a slow, continuous injection over an extended timeframe (**Fig. 4**).

Complications of embolization include discoloration of overlying skin, with agents such as aetoxisclerol and Onyx. Tattooing and extrusion scarring can occur after Onyx use, leading to this discoloration. Other agents such as ethanol and cyanoacrylate (bioadhesive) can extrude and cause localized inflammation and toxicity.[22]

Laser Therapy

Endovenous laser therapy diode at 980 nm; 5 to 8 W; 1470 at 8 W.
 Fiber 400 to 600 μm.
 Power setting at 300 J/cm^2

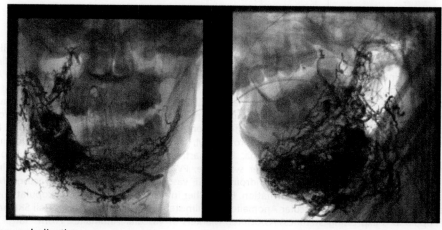

Fig. 4. Onyx embolization.

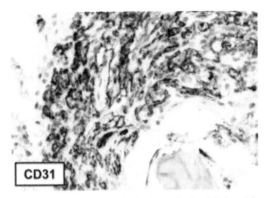

Fig. 5. IHC showing endothelial cells highlighted by CD31.

Energy 8 to 12 W for deep lesions and 3 to 5 W for superficial lesions.

250 to 300 J/cm^3.

Medical Treatments

Doxycycline has been used in arteriovenous malformations and hurriedly hemorrhagic telangiectasia. Common epistaxis associated with HHT is treated with doxycycline. In addition, anti-inflammatory and antiangiogenic agents, such as interferon,

reduce matrix metallic proteinase-9 and inhibit pro-inflammatory cytokines.[23]

Sirolimus, the first inhibitor of mTOR, was discovered in the 1970s as part of a screening program for new antifungal agents and was first named rapamycin because it was isolated from a soil sample from Rapa Nui.[24] It was not until the 1990s that it was developed as an immunosuppressant, used mainly for allograft rejection based on its ability to interrupt the complex intracellular signaling cascade of the mTOR pathway.

Treatment of Gorham–Stout Disease

There are no definitive therapy recommendations for GSD. Radiation therapy has been used to successfully prevent GSD progression, typically at lower doses of 30 to 45 Gy. Although radiation may arrest endothelial cell proliferation, it increases the risk of developing sarcoma and secondary malignancy.[17,18]

Anti-vascular and immunosuppressant medications have shown effectiveness in slowing and even reversing the affected sites of GSD. Those medications target the lymphatic vessels that grow abnormally and disrupt the body's normal bone regeneration process. Sirolimus, as mentioned above, is an oral immunosuppressant

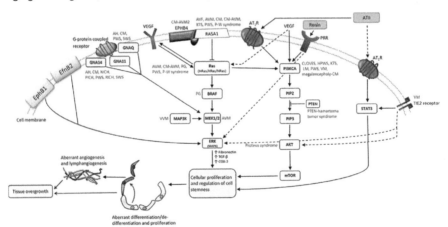

Fig. 6. A proposed model for the role of gene mutations involving the Ras/BRAF/MEK/ERK and the PI3KCA/AKT/mTOR pathways by their interaction with different components of the renin-angiotensin system, leading to the induction and/or maintenance of cells that express stemness-associated markers in vascular anomalies. AH, anastomosing hemangioma; AT1R, angiotensin II receptor 1; AT2R, angiotensin II receptor 2; ATII, angiotensin II; AVF, arteriovenous fistula; AVM, arteriovenous malformation; CLOVES, congenital lipomatous overgrowth with vascular–epidermal and skeletal anomalies; CM, capillary malformation; CM-AVM, capillary malformation-arteriovenous malformation; CM-AVM2, capillary malformation-arteriovenous malformation 2; HPWS, hypertrophic port-wine stain; KTS, Klippel–Trénaunay syndrome; LM, lymphatic malformation; NICH, non-involuting congenital hemangioma; PG, pyogenic granuloma; PICH, partially involuting congenital hemangioma; PRR, pro-renin receptor; P-W syndrome, Parkes–Weber syndrome; PWS, port-wine stain; RICH, rapidly involuting congenital hemangioma; SWS, Sturge–Weber syndrome; VEGF, vascular endothelial growth factor; VM, venous malformation; VVM, verrucous venous malformation. For further information refer to "Cell Populations Expressing Stemness-Associated Markers in Vascular Anomalies".[1] (Kilmister EJ, Hansen L, Davis PF, Hall SRR and Tan ST (2021) Cell Populations Expressing Stemness-Associated Markers in Vascular Anomalies. Front. Surg. 7:610758. https://doi.org/10.3389/fsurg.2020.610758.)

Table 1
Overview of vascular tumors of bone

		Hemangioma	Epithelioid Hemangioma	Pseudomyogenic Hemangioendothelioma	Epithelioid Hemangioendothelioma	Angiosarcoma
Biological Potential		Benign	Intermediate-locally aggressive	Intermediate-rarely metastasizing	Malignant	
Clinical features	Prevalence	Common (~10%)		Rare (≤1 in 1,000,000)		
	Percentage of patients with multifocal presentation	<20	~20	>90	>50	>50
	Percentage 5-y overall survival	100		>95	~75	<40
Radiographic features		Lytic ("corduroy like")		Lytic to mixed lytic-sclerotic		Lytic and aggressive
Histologic features	Border	Smooth	Smooth	Infiltrative and ragged	Infiltrative and ragged	Infiltrative and ragged
	Lobulation	Yes	Yes	No	No	No
	Vasoformation	Yes	Yes	No	Usually no[a]	Variable
	Cytologic features	Spindled	Epithelioid	Spindled-to-epithelioid	Epithelioid-to-spindled	
	Necrosis	Uncommon	Occasional	Occasional	Occasional	Frequent
Immunohistochemistry	Cytokeratins	None		Positive in a subset of all vascular tumors		
	Diagnostic markers for distinction	None	FOSB (in a subset of tumors)	FOSB	CAMTA1 (rarely TFE3)	None
Recurrent genetic mutations		None	FOS (rarely FOSB rearrangement)	FOSB rearrangement	WWTR1-CAMTA1 (rarely YAP1-TFE3 or other) fusion	Diverse

[a] Although most epithelioid hemangioendotheliomas lack vasoformative features, well-formed vascular channels are present in a small subset of tumors (that harbor the YAP1-TFE3 fusion).

Adapted from Hung YP. Vascular Tumors of Bone: Updates and Diagnostic Pitfall. Surg Pathol Clin. 2021 Dec;14(4):645-663.[1]

medication that targets lymphatic vessel formation. It can generally stabilize the disease and effectively slow the progression of GSD while reducing symptoms and complications. Recent studies have shown clinical benefit with stability of imaging findings. Interferon-alpha-2 also inhibits the formation of lymphatic vessels and has been noted to improve symptoms. Bisphosphonates work to slow bone loss, which can help stabilize GSD, though most physicians consider GSD is a proliferation of vessels instead of an osteoclastic disease.

Surgical treatment is recommended for pathologic fractures or reconstruction of massively destroyed bone. Surgery alone cannot cure GSD, but physicians may recommend surgical procedures to stabilize or remove affected bone or to treat symptoms and complications related to the disease. Surgery outcomes are improved when the disease is concurrently managed medically.

Interventional radiology procedures with bleomycin along with or cyanoacrylate-based intraosseous injections may block progression of bone loss. This is assumable with antiangiogenic activity of bleomycin and fibrous scarring within residual bone tissue. The combination of bleomycin and cyanoacrylate, especially in the non-weight-bearing facial skeleton such as the zygoma, can prevent gross asymmetry.[23] Bleomycin is reconstituted in appropriate weighted units using normal saline, mixed 1:1 with 25% albumin and air, to create a foam. Intraoperative ultrasound guidance can be enhanced by using add 1 cc of Ethiodol for visualization on imaging. Pre-operative embolization is commonly performed under fluoroscopy with a n-butyl cyanoacrylate/Ethiodol mixture, flushing needles with dextrose 5% in water. Follow-up imaging can assess the embolization with computed tomorgraphy, magnetic resonance imaging, or conebeam CT.[18]

GENETIC FACTORS

Vascular markers such as ERG, FLI1, CD34, CD30, and CD31 are used to highlight endothelial cells (**Fig. 5**). Fragments of endothelial cells are adequate for diagnosis of a vascular tumor of bone unless it is a high-flow AVM. Mutations in FOS, FOSB, WWTR1-CAMTA1, or YAP1-TFE3 fusion have also been reported.[1] EWSR1-NFATC1 molecular fusion gene has been reported in 22 q 12 chromosome band. EWSR1 chimera has been associated with spectrum of neoplasms including Ewing sarcoma.[2]

Mutations that involve the Ras/BRAF/MEK/ERK and the PI3KCA/AKT/mTOR pathways, via interaction with the renin-angiotensin system, can lead to cellular expression of cancer stem-cell markers in vascular anomalies (**Fig. 6**). Testing for PIK3CA mutations can be considered if vascular malformations such as large capillary, lymphatic, or venous malformations are found. The PIK3CA-related overgrowth spectrum is a broad-ranging spectrum of disorders caused by PIK3CA mutations, involving overgrowth of adipose, muscle, nerve, or skeletal tissue, vascular or lymphatic malformations, and skin lesions.

The foundation of cellular growth and replication is established by the PI3K/Akt/mTOR pathway. In addition, it enhances the production of vascular endothelial growth factor (VEGF), thereby governing the processes of angiogenesis and lymphangiogenesis. Inhibitors of mTOR act by directly restraining mTOR activity, which subsequently hampers the synthesis of proteins further down the signaling cascade.[22] As a result, these inhibitors exhibit both antitumor and antiangiogenic effects and represent targeted therapy for those conditions affected by PI3K/Akt/mTOR pathway mutations. RASopathies are a cluster of anomalies due to activation of the RAS–MAPK signaling with germline changes. These mosaic-like pathogenic variations may be responsible for some lymphatic anomalies.

Genetic testing can be performed for most patients and can guide therapy and provide insight to pathogenesis. Some diseases have specific genotype to phenotype correlations, whereas some are more nonspecific in presentation such as the PIK3CA associated anomalies. Some of the mutations that have been identified are somatic mutations that can be assessed by obtaining affected tissue. PCR-based assays of the specific mutations can be conducted in a similar fashion to oncological conditions. Mosaic conditions need tissue samples from the affected tissue and deep sequencing can be performed. Further, as many of these anomalies are part of syndromes, other tissue specimens or whole blood might become necessary for comparison. Finally, studying the proliferation of cells with vascular mutations will aid in the development of future therapies.

SUMMARY

Management of maxillofacial vascular anomalies remains challenging. Diagnosis is paramount to determining the correct treatment modality and preventing disease progression. The development of early screening methods and risk stratification criteria may eventually assist with treatment. Advances have been made in our understanding of genetic pathways that are linked to vascular tumors and malformations as well as adjacent diseases such as Gorham-Stout Disease (GSD).

GSD is a rare entity of unknown etiopathology characterized by destruction of osseous matrix, proliferation of lymphatic vascular structures, and massive regional osteolysis. The diagnosis is made by exclusion of other diseases, particularly other vascular or lymphatic diseases, such as lymphangioma or angiosarcoma. To establish a diagnosis, evaluation of histologic, radiological, and clinical features are critical.

CLINICS CARE POINTS

- Diagnosis is key when treating vascular anomalies, and terminology can often be misleading. Irrespective of the diagnosis (i.e., malformation or tumor), thorough phenotyping and an understanding of biologic behavior are paramount for developing patient-specific therapies.

- Magnetic resonance imaging with contrast is the gold-standard for diagnostic workup of a craniofacial vascular lesion.

- Gorham-Stout Disease is a rare disorder and a diagnosis of exclusion. It should be considered in the differential when massive osteolysis is present in one or more adjacent bones.

- Advances in the molecular genetics of vascular lesions, particularly into the understanding of the Ras/BRAF/MEK/ERK and the PI3KCA/AKT/mTOR pathways, may provide critical insights into etiology and future treatment.

FUNDING

This manuscript was supported in part by the Laborator for Applied Clinical Research and Research and Training Fund, Department of Oral & Maxillofacial Surgery, University of Washington School of Dentistry.

DISCLOSURES

The authors have no disclosures.

REFERENCES

1. Hung YP. Vascular Tumors of Bone: Updates and Diagnostic Pitfall. Surg Pathol Clin 2021;14(4):645–63.
2. Arbajian E, Magnusson L, Brosjo O, et al. A benign vascular tumor with a new fusion gene: EWSR1-NFATC1 in hemangioma of the bone. Am J Surg Pathol 2013;37:613–6.
3. Kaban LB, Troulis MJ. Pediatric oral and maxillofacial surgery. Philadelphia: WB Saunders; 2004.
4. Mulliken JB, Glowacki J. Hemangiomas and vascular malformations in infants and children: a classification based on endothelial characteristics. Plast Reconstr Surg 1982;69(3):412–22.
5. Mulliken JB, Young AE. Vascular birthmarks: hemangiomas and malformations. Philadelphia: WB Saunders; 1988.
6. Jackson JBS. A boneless arm. Boston Med Surg J 1838;18:368–9.
7. Gorham LW, Stout AP. Massive osteolysis (acute spontaneous absorption of bone, phantom bone, disappearing bone): its relation to hemangiomatosis. J Bone Joint Surg [Am] 1955;37-A:985–1004.
8. Wright IS. Memorial. L. Whittington Gorham, M.D. Trans Am Clin Climatol Assoc 1969;80:xlvii–xlviii.
9. Lattes R. In memoriam- Arthur Purdy Stout, M.D. (1885-1967). Am J Clin Pathol 1968;50:251–2.
10. Heyden G, Kindblom LG, Nielsen JM. Disappearing bone disease. A clinical and histological study. J Bone Joint Surg Am 1977;59(1):57–61.
11. Young JW, Galbraith M, Cunningham J, et al. Progressive vertebral collapse in diffuse angiomatosis. Metab Bone Dis Relat Res 1983;5(2):53–60.
12. Momanu A, Caba L, Gorduza NC, et al. Gorham-Stout Disease with Multiple Bone Involvement—Challenging Diagnosis of a Rare Disease and Literature Review. Medicina 2021;57(7):681.
13. Heffez L, Doku HC, Carter BL, et al. Perspectives on massive osteolysis. Report of a case and review of the literature. Oral Surg Oral Med Oral Pathol 1983;55:331–43.
14. Gorham-Stout Disease | Boston Children's Hospital. www.childrenshospital.org. https://www.childrenshospital.org/conditions/gorham-stout-disease#:~:text=Children%20with%20Gorham%2DStout%20disease.
15. Zheng C, Tang F, Min L, et al. Gorham-Stout disease of the malleolus: a rare case report. BMC Muscoskel Disord 2020;21(1). https://doi.org/10.1186/s12891-019-3027-9.
16. Chung C, Yu JS, Resnick D, et al. Gorham syndrome of the thorax and cervical spine: CT and MRI findings. Skeletal Radiol 1997;26(1):55–9.
17. Rodriguez-Vazquez JR, Chandra SR, Albertson ME, et al. Radiation-Induced Sarcoma on 18F-FDG PET/CT After Treatment of Gorham-Stout Disease of the Maxilla. Clin Nucl Med 2019;44(11):e607–8.
18. Nair SC, Chandra SR. Management of head and neck vascular lesions: a guide for surgeons. 1st edition. Springer Nature, Singapore; 2022.
19. Liu Y, Zhong D-R, Zhou P-R, et al. Gorham-Stout disease: radiological, histological, and clinical features of 12 cases and review of literature. Clin Rheumatol 2016;35(3):813–23.
20. Heyd R, Micke O, Surholt C, et al. Radiation Therapy for Gorham-Stout Syndrome: Results of a National Patterns-of-Care Study and Literature Review. Int J Radiat Oncol Biol Phys 2011;81(3):e179–85.

21. Ganau M, Syrmos NC, D'Arco F, et al. Enhancing contrast agents and radiotracers performance through hyaluronic acid-coating in neuroradiology and nuclear medicine. Hell J Nucl Med 2017;20(2): 166–8.

22. Forero Saldarriaga S, Vallejo C, Urrea Pineda L, et al. Gorham-Stout Disease with Clinical Response to Sirolimus Treatment. European Journal of Case Reports in Internal Medicine 2021. https://doi.org/10.12890/2021_002740.

23. Wang W, Yeung KWK. Bone grafts and biomaterials substitutes for bone defect repair: A review. Bioact Mater 2017;2(4):224–47.

24. Hartford CM, Ratain MJ. Rapamycin: something old, something new, sometimes borrowed and now renewed. Clin Pharmacol Ther 2007;82(4):381–8.

Medical Management of Nonmalignant Vascular Tumors of the Head and Neck
Part 1

Jorie Gatts, MD[a], Srinivasa Chandra, MD[b], Deepak Krishnan, DDS[c,d], Kiersten Ricci, MD[a,d],*

KEYWORDS

- Infantile hemangioma • Congenital hemangioma • Kaposiform hemangioendothelioma
- Propranolol • Timolol • Sirolimus

KEY POINTS

- First-line treatment of complicated infantile hemangiomas is with the beta-adrenergic antagonist, oral propranolol.
- Topical timolol can be considered for less complicated superficial infantile hemangiomas.
- Kaposiform hemangioendothelioma (KHE) is a locally aggressive vascular tumor that is associated with a life-threatening coagulopathy, Kasabach–Merritt phenomenon (KMP). Early consultation with hematology/oncology for management is critical.
- Complete excision of KHE is curative but may not be feasible if KMP is present or the tumor is extensive and infiltrative across tissue and fascial planes.
- KHE with KMP requires urgent treatment with medical therapeutics such as sirolimus and may require embolization for temporalization.

INTRODUCTION

Vascular anomalies (VAs), broadly classified as nonmalignant tumors and malformations, consist of a multitude of disorders that have a wide range of symptoms and complications as well as overlapping clinical, radiologic, and histologic findings. Distinguishing between non-malignant vascular tumors and malformations, as well as the precise diagnosis within these distinctions, is critical because prognosis, therapy, and chronicity of care vary greatly. In contrast to normal endothelial turnover in vascular malformations, vascular tumors are characterized by the abnormal proliferation of endothelial cells and aberrant blood vessels.

Nonmalignant vascular tumors including infantile and congenital hemangiomas and kaposiform hemangioendothelioma (KHE) frequently affect the head and neck area. Proliferative masses in the head and neck area can cause substantial morbidity and can be life-threatening. Potential complications of head and neck vascular tumors include airway obstruction, vision and hearing impairment, facial disfigurement, infection, coagulopathy, bleeding, and feeding and speech

[a] Hemangioma and Vascular Malformation Center, Cancer and Blood Diseases Institute, Cincinnati Children's Hospital Medical Center, 3333 Burnet Avenue, MLC 7015, Cincinnati, OH 45229, USA; [b] Department of Oral and Maxillofacial Surgery–Head and Neck Oncology and Microvascular Reconstruction, Oregon Health and Sciences University, 3181 SW Sam Jackson Park Road, Portland, OR 97239, USA; [c] Department of Surgery, Section of Oral & Maxillofacial Surgery, University of Cincinnati, 200 Albert Sabin Way, ML 0461, Cincinnati, OH 45219, USA; [d] University of Cincinnati College of Medicine, 231 Albert Sabin Way, Cincinnati, OH 45267-0558, USA
* Corresponding author. Division of Hematology, Cancer and Blood Diseases Institute, Cincinnati Children's Hospital Medical Center, 3333 Burnet Avenue, MLC 7015, Cincinnati, Ohio 45229
E-mail address: Kiersten.Ricci@cchmc.org

Oral Maxillofacial Surg Clin N Am 36 (2024) 103–113
https://doi.org/10.1016/j.coms.2023.09.011
1042-3699/24/© 2023 Elsevier Inc. All rights reserved.

issues as well as psychosocial and economic stressors.

In the past, medical therapy options for nonmalignant and intermediate, or locally aggressive, vascular tumors were insufficient. Intralesional, oral, and topical corticosteroids were the primary medical options for treatment of infantile hemangiomas, and side effects with long-term use can be detrimental, particularly in infants and young children. Despite the lack of scientific evidence of safety and efficacy, many drugs, including chemotherapeutic agents, were historically used in the attempt to control, typically with varied or inadequate response, the aggressive nature of KHE, an intermediate tumor associated with the severe coagulopathy and significant morbidity.

Recently, medical therapeutics, including propranolol, timolol, and sirolimus, have changed the paradigm in the treatment of benign and intermediate vascular tumors. The serendipitous discovery of the efficaciousness of beta-adrenergic blockage, specifically with oral propranolol, revolutionized the treatment paradigm for infantile hemangiomas.[1] Oral propranolol quickly became first-line therapy and substantially lessened the need for interventions such as surgical excision and laser therapy.

In a patient KHE with severe Kasabach–Merritt phenomenon (KMP) and multiorgan failure who had failed all previous treatments including steroids, vincristine, cyclophosphamide, bevacizumab, and embolization therapy, oral sirolimus was first used, in the compassionate care setting, and found to have remarkable efficacy.[2,3] Because of this success, despite the consensus-driven 2013 recommendations for upfront treatment with vincristine and steroids, systemic sirolimus, often in combination with corticosteroids and with or without vincristine, has emerged as the primary treatment for KHE with KMP. Complete surgical excision is curative, but if often not possible. Embolization of problematic arterial feeding vessels remains an important temporizing measure in initial care.

VASCULAR TUMORS

Vascular tumors are characterized by the abnormal proliferation of endothelial cells and aberrant blood vessels. Vascular tumors are classified as benign, locally aggressive (intermediate), or malignant. In the head and neck area, these tumors can be life-threatening, disfiguring, or cause significant functional impairment. Previously, corticosteroids and traditional chemotherapeutic agents were used as single agents or as adjuncts to surgical interventions when treating vascular tumors. However, these medical therapies have variable efficacy and numerous well-known short- and long-term adverse effects. More recently, the efficacy of propranolol, timolol, and sirolimus has been recognized. Excluding malignancy, this section concentrates on benign and locally aggressive vascular tumors including hemangiomas and KHE.

Infantile Hemangioma

Natural course/diagnosis
Infantile hemangiomas (IHs) are the most common tumor in children, occurring in approximately 5% of infants.[4] IHs are benign vascular growths, primarily consisting of capillaries and proliferating endothelial cells. IHs occur on all areas of the body but are common in the head and neck area.[5] IHs are more likely to occur with prematurity, multiple births (twins, triplets, and so forth), advanced maternal age, and placental complications.[5–7]

Although IHs are typically not proliferating at birth, a precursor lesion, such as an area of pallor, telangiectasia, or pink-red or purple macule or patch, may be identifiable. If not recognized at or near time of birth, most IHs are apparent by 3 to 8 weeks, although this is variable depending on the size, morphology, and location of the lesion(s). Generally, IHs proliferate for approximately 4 to 6 months, followed by slow involution over several years for complete resolution.[8] However, IHs can have a longer proliferation phase lasting until 2 to 3 years of age, especially when involving the airway, nose, parotid space, or orbital area and may not completely resolve.

Most IHs can be diagnosed by history and physical examination. Rarely, atypical features or presentation necessitate a biopsy. Histologically, IHs characteristically stain positive for endothelial glucose transporter 1 (GLUT1) during all phases of their natural course[9]; GLUT1 is also expressed on placental endothelial cells but absent in other vascular malformations and most other vascular tumors.[10] During the proliferative phase, pro-vasculogenic factors, such as vascular endothelial growth factor, basic fibroblast growth factor, CD34, and CD31 are also expressed.[5,7,11]

Treatment
Most uncomplicated IHs do not require treatment, and watchful observation, along with anticipatory guidance, is recommended. However, in patients with complicated IH and those in high-risk anatomic sites, such as the head and neck, early consultation with a hemangioma specialist, ideally by 1 to 2 months of age, is critical to facilitate treatment and prevent adverse outcomes. Complications of IHs involving the head and neck are common and can result in physical deformity,

hearing loss, vision impairment, and respiratory issues. Orbital, mucosal, airway, and maxillofacial IHs, particularly those with rapid growth, can cause significant ulceration, bleeding, pain, secondary infection, significant anatomic asymmetry, and psychological effects on the child.[5,6] Many of these infants need urgent inpatient care to address wound issues, treatment of infection, and medication initiation, along with evaluation for airway or vascular syndromic correlations. Importantly, treatment should not only be initiated with the development of acute issues but should also be considered early for the prevention of short-term and long-term complications. More than one-half of children with untreated hemangiomas experience residual changes such as scarring, atrophy, redundant skin, discoloration, telangiectasia, or fibroadipose tissue, which is an important consideration for head and neck IHs.[12]

Beta-adrenergic inhibitors, including propranolol and timolol, have overwhelmingly emerged as first-line therapy for IHs. The effectiveness of propranolol in the treatment of IHs was discovered serendipitously in 2008 when the medication was used in infants with cardiac disease, and their IHs had notably smaller sizes and earlier regression.[1] Since then, two randomized control trials have demonstrated the safety and efficacy of propranolol for treatment of IHs, with an estimated treatment failure rate of only 1% to 2%.[8,13,14] In addition to both clinical trials demonstrating non-inferiority of propranolol to systemic corticosteroids, propranolol was better tolerated with fewer side effects.[15,16] An oral formation of propranolol specifically for the treatment of IHs was approved by the US Food and Drug Administration (FDA) in 2014.

Oral propranolol is typically initiated at doses of 0.5 to 1 mg/kg/day, divided in two to three doses per day and escalated to 2 to 3 mg/kg/day. In infants, propranolol is generally well tolerated with few significant side effects.[4] The most concerning potential side effects include hypoglycemia, bradycardia, and hypotension, though these can typically be avoided by increasing the dose incrementally, monitoring closely, and holding doses before anticipated fasting states or with decreased oral intake due to illness.[13] Caution should be exercised in neonates (<5 weeks of age), premature infants, and infants with known cardiovascular, cerebrovascular, and/or pulmonary disease and should be evaluated by the appropriate subspecialists prior to starting propranolol.[4] Other oral beta-blockers, such as atenolol and nadolol, have also been used to treat IH but less clinical data are available.[17,18] One prospective study of 27 children found that atenolol, a selective beta −1 antagonist, was non-inferior to propranolol for treatment of IHs.[19] Although it has been suggested that atenolol may have less risk of side effects such as bronchospasm, given its selective beta-adrenergic inhibition, this has not been studied prospectively to date. However, its use is intriguing in individuals with IHs and concurrent cerebrovascular abnormalities because atenolol is hydrophilic and therefore, less likely to cross the blood-brain barrier.

Topical timolol maleate has become a favored treatment in less aggressive IHs because of the lower potential for serious side effects. Although timolol is currently not an approved FDA treatment for IHs, the medication is readily available as an ophthalmic preparation in a solution or gel formulation, which can both be directly applied to IHs; multiple concentrations of the solution and gel are available but the 0.5% concentation is mostly commonly used and studied. Multiple studies have revealed that timolol is effective in diminishing the color, size, and volume, particularly when used in the rapid proliferative phase of superficial IHs.[20–22] Local skin irritation is the most common side effect, although still rare. When used as prescribed, any systemic absorption does not seem clinically relevant.[23] One study suggested that adverse events are more likely to occur in infants who are less than 1 month adjusted age, weigh less than 2500 g, or have a history of prematurity, apnea, or bradycardia.[24] The risk of side effects also increases with timolol application at sites of high absorption such as in or near the eye, intertriginous areas, and mucosal and ulcerated surfaces. Standardized dosing of topical timolol for IHs has not been established to date.

While effective, corticosteroids are no longer the first-line treatment for IHs, but may be used in conjunction with oral propranolol to achieve a quicker initial response or when beta-blockers are contraindicated or ineffective.[6] Multiple studies have reported effectiveness of intralesional steroid as treatment for IHs, but this has been mostly used for well-localized lesions causing increased bulk and distortion of anatomic landmarks such as the lip.[4] Because safety and efficacy of steroid injections is limited to few applicable IHs, along with the need for anesthesia and often multiple procedures, this modality has clinically fallen out of favor in the United States, particularly since oral propranolol is commercially available. In the rare situations in which IHs have failed conventional therapies or when beta-blockers are contraindicated, sirolimus has been used given its antiproliferative and antiangiogenic effects demonstrated in vitro studies of hemangioma endothelial cells.[25–27]

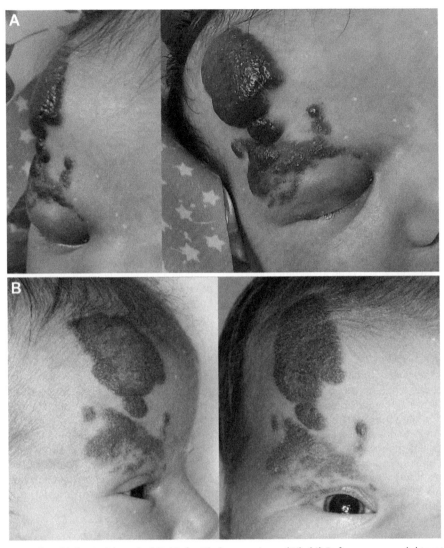

Fig. 1. Photographs of infant with periorbital infantile hemangioma (IH). (*A*) Before propranolol treatment. Due to involvement of the upper eyelid, the infant was unable to open the eye and had complete visual obstruction. (*B*) One month on propranolol treatment. Infant has significant decrease in IH of upper eyelid and now able to open eye with only mild ptosis.

Duration of treatment for IHs varies based on the size and location. Because IHs typically have growth potential for 6 to 9 months, treatment is generally extended to 9 to 12 months to avoid rebound growth. Rebound growth is a known potential complication with cessation of treatment, and some patients may need to be restarted on propranolol. Topical timolol may be used to treat mild to moderate regrowth. Although the pathophysiology is not understood, IHs of the head and neck, particularly those involving the airway, nose, periorbital/orbital area, and parotid gland, often require treatment for 2 or 3 years to avoid rebound growth as well as to achieve the best results with medication alone.

Periorbital/orbital infantile hemangioma

Periorbital and orbital IHs can cause visual compromise. Most commonly, eyelid IHs, when large enough, can cause ptosis and obstruct the visual axis, which not only causes acute partial or complete vision obstruction of the affected eye but can also lead to long-term complications such as stimulus-deprivation amblyopia and strabismus. Subcutaneous IHs in the periocular area can extend into the orbit and result in proptosis/exophthalmos, globe displacement, and/or increased intraocular pressure.[28] Computed tomography and/or MRI with and without contrast are recommended for IHs at high risk for deeper orbital involvement. All periorbital and orbital IHs,

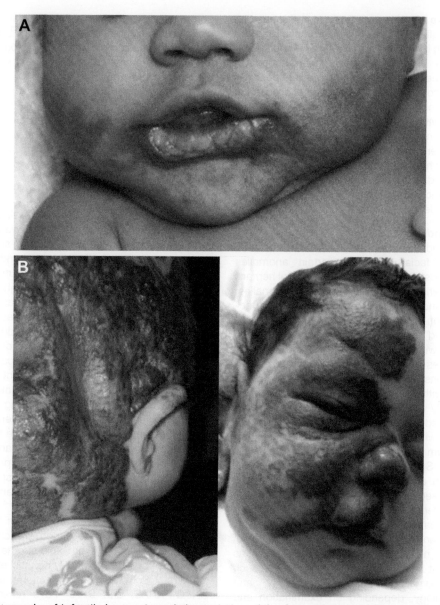

Fig. 2. Photographs of infantile hemangioma (IH) associations. (*A*) Infant with IH involving the chin, lower lip, and jawline in a "bearded" distribution. Subglottic hemangioma was found on endoscopy. (*B*) Infants with large segmental IH on the scalp and neck, and the other on the face. Both infants were discovered to have other abnormalities meeting criteria for PHACE syndrome.

as well as those with any possibility of potential visual impairment, should have an ophthalmologic evaluation. For individuals with visual obstruction, treatment with propranolol, typically at dosing of 3 mg/kg/day has been effective (**Fig. 1**).[4,29] Intraocular timolol has been used to treat orbital IHs; a combination of intraocular and topical timolol has also been used to manageeyelid IHs.[30] Intraocular use of timolol should be done in consultation with ophthalmology and generally should not exceed twice daily dosing in the eye or on the

thin skin of the eyelid. Lagophthalmos due to proptosis with orbital IHs can be surgically treated for symptom management along with medical therapy. Wall decompression and moisture chambers with canthopexy can be performed.

Airway infantile hemangioma

Segmental IHs involving the anterior neck, chin, lower lip, and jawline, particularly in a "bearded" distribution (**Fig. 2**A) are at risk for associated airway IHs. However, subglottic IHs may occur in the absence of cutaneous findings.[31] Because of the small caliber of the airway in an infant, rapidly proliferating IHs can lead to life-threatening airway obstruction. Flexible nasopharyngeal endoscopy should be performed by a maxillofacial specialist or otolaryngologist for complete evaluation for subglottic IHs and other lesions in the airway. Systemic treatment with propranolol at dosing of 3 mg/kg/day is first-line therapy for airway IHs.[4] Concurrent use of systemic corticosteroid is also a consideration for symptomatic obstructive lesions causing respiratory distress. Sclerotherapy, surgery, laser ablation, and intralesional steroid are also treatment considerations, but second or third line.[32]

PHACE syndrome

PHACE syndrome is an association of cutaneous segmental facial IHs with certain anomalies including posterior fossa anomalies, facial hemangioma, arterial abnormalities, cardiac anomalies, and eye abnormalities (see **Fig. 2**B).[33] A prospective study of 108 infants with large facial hemangiomas found that 31% of patients had findings consistent with PHACE syndrome.[33] The spectrum of anomalies in PHACE syndrome suggests that a causative insult likely occurs in the first trimester, probably within the first 3 to 12 weeks of gestation during early vasculogenesis. PHACE syndrome is now believed to be predominantly a congenital vasculopathy with multiple features occurring due to downstream events of arteriopathy and resultant ischemia.[4] Specific diagnostic criteria for PHACE association are published (**Table 1**).[34,35] Infants with large segmental IHs on the face and/or scalp should undergo evaluation with physical examination, echocardiogram, ophthalmologic examination, MRI, and magnetic resonance angiogram of the head, neck, and mediastinum as well as assessment by any pertinent subspecialties such as neurosurgery, neurology, cardiology, and otolaryngology, depending on examination and testing results. IHs of the internal auditory canal can be associated with hearing loss and should be assessed.[4,36] If cerebrovascular or cardiovascular abnormalities are present, consultation with neurology and cardiology is advised before initiation of propranolol.[6] As previously mentioned, atenolol may be a treatment option given its hydrophilic nature with less likely crossing of the blood-brain barrier.

Congenital Hemangioma

Congenital hemangiomas (CHs) are benign vascular tumors that are clinically and biologically different than IHs. CHs are fully developed before birth and most often located on the head, neck, or extremities. Although CHs do not grow after birth, some may rapidly involute or partially involute over weeks to months or even years.[37] Although CHs can occasionally appear histologically like IHs, CHs are characteristically GLUT-1 negative.[38] Oral propranolol and topical timolol are not beneficial in the treatment of CHs. If a lesion is painful, functionally limiting, or is persistently ulcerated or bleeding, surgical excision is indicated. Pulsed-dye laser for skin discoloration and embolization for significant arteriovenous shunting in large CHs are also management considerations.[39]

Pyogenic Granuloma

Pyogenic granulomas (PGs), also called lobular capillary hemangiomas, are benign vascular tumors characterized by rapid growth and friable surface, typically affecting the skin and mucous membranes at sites of prior tissue injury or overlying a capillary malformation. Although most are solitary lesions, PGs can present as multiple grouped (also called "eruptive") or disseminated tumors (**Fig. 3**). PGs occur in individuals of all ages and are common in children. Although spontaneous resolution is possible, PGs can regrow and frequently bleed without treatment. Surgical excision is the most common treatment as it has the lowest rate of recurrence.[40] Curettage, electrocautery, radiosurgery, cryosurgery, sclerotherapy, or laser treatment are other alternative treatment options depending on the area, size, and patient preferences.[41] Topical timolol and oral propranolol have been reported to be beneficial in specific circumstances including pediatric (children <9 years of age), periungual, and ocular PGs.[42–44]

Histologically, PGs are composed of capillaries and venules with plump endothelial cells separated into lobules by fibromyxoid stroma and stain negatively for GLUT-1 and lymphatic endothelial markers.[41] Somatic gain-of-function mutations in GNAQ, KRAS, and BRAF have recently been linked to the etiology of pyogenic granuloma.[45] Overactivation of the RAS/MAPK pathway suggests that BRAF and/or MEK inhibition may be beneficial in complicated PGs such as those that are disseminated, located on difficult-to-treat mucosal surfaces, or recur despite multiple surgical interventions. Topical MEK inhibitor, trametinib, is commercially available in the United States and is also a treatment consideration. Although topical BRAF inhibitor is currently not commercially available, it is currently being studied in other dermatologic conditions.

Kaposiform Hemangioendothelioma

Kaposiform hemangioendothelioma (KHE) is a locally aggressive vascular tumor that, although

Table 1
PHACE syndrome criteria

Definite PHACE	Possible PHACE
Hemangioma >5 cm in diameter of the head including scalp PLUS 1 major criteria or 2 minor criteria Hemangioma of the neck, upper trunk or trunk and proximal upper extremity PLUS 2 major criteria	Hemangioma >5 cm in diameter of the head including scalp PLUS 1 minor criteria Hemangioma of the neck, upper trunk or trunk and proximal upper extremity PLUS 1 major or 2 minor No hemangioma PLUS 2 major criteria

Body System	Major Criteria	Minor Criteria
Brain	• Posterior fossa brain anomalies • Dandy-Walker complex • Other hypoplasia/dysplasia of the mid and/or hindbrain	• Midline brain anomalies • Malformation of cortical development
Cardiovascular	• Aortic arch anomalies • Coarctation of the aorta • Dysplasia[a] • Aneurysm • Aberrant origin of the subclavian artery with or without a vascular ring	• Ventricular septal defect • Right aortic arch/double aortic arch • Systemic venous anomalies
Cerebrovascular	• Anomaly of major cerebral or cervical arteries[b] • Dysplasia of the large cerebral or cervical arteries[a] • Arterial stenosis or occlusion with or without moyamoya collaterals Absence or moderate–severe hypoplasia of the large cerebral and cervical arteries • Aberrant origin or course of the large cerebral or cervical arteries except common arch variants such as bovine arch • Persistent carotid-vertebrobasilar anastomosis (proatlantal segmental, hypoglossal, otic, and/or trigeminal arteries)	• Aneurysm of any of the cerebral arteries
Eye	• Posterior segment abnormalities • Persistent hyperplastic primary vitreous • Persistent fetal vasculature • Retinal vascular anomalies • Morning glory disc anomaly • Optic nerve hypoplasia • Peripapillary staphyloma	• Anterior segment abnormalities • Microphthalmia • Sclerocornea • Coloboma • Cataracts
Midline/Ventral	• Anomaly of the midline chest and abdomen • Sternal defect • Sternal pit • Sternal cleft • Supraumbilical raphe	• Ectopic thyroid hypopituitarism • Midline sternal papule/hamartoma

[a] Includes kinking, looping, tortuosity, and/or dolichoectasia.
[b] Internal carotid artery, middle cerebral artery, anterior cerebral artery, posterior cerebral artery, or vertebrobasilar system.
Adapted from Garzon and colleagues.[35]

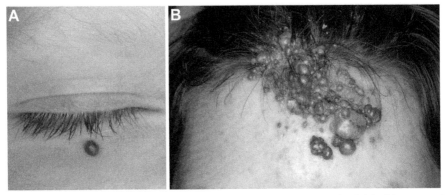

Fig. 3. Photographs with two children with pyogenic granulomas (PGs). (*A*) Male child with uncomplicated solitary lesion. (*B*) Adolescent female with multiple grouped or "eruptive" PGs.

rare, is associated with high morbidity. Classically, KHE presents in infancy or early childhood as a solitary tumor that is frequently warm, indurated, and red or purple in color; however, lesions can appear ill-defined and purpuric or be located completely internally.[46,47] Although KHE may occur on any body part, the head, neck, and extremities are common. Diagnosis can be challenging due to clinical heterogeneity and nonspecific imaging findings that overlap with other benign and malignant vascular tumors, including CHs and angiosarcoma (**Fig. 4**).[48,49] Thus, biopsy is often instrumental in diagnosis. Histologically, KHE is composed of coalescing nodules of spindle (kaposiform) and epithelioid cells and expresses lymphatic endothelial markers, podoplanin (D2–40), and PROX-1; KHE is GLUT-1 negative.[50] Tufted angioma (TA), a

less aggressive tumor, can have similar histology but is generally confined to the superficial tissues, whereas KHE is often infiltrative, crossing tissue/fascial planes and even extending into the thoracic or abdominal cavities or bone, including the mandible. KHE tumors may cause pain, intermittent enlargement, functional limitations, skin discoloration or purpura, physical deformity, and psychosocial distress. With suspected or confirmed KHE, early consultation with a hematologist/oncologist is highly recommended.

The most serious complication of KHE is the development of a life-threatening coagulopathy called Kasabach-Merritt phenomenon (KMP), which is characterized by severe thrombocytopenia and hypofibrinogenemia.[51] KMP is estimated to occur in approximately 60% to 70% of KHE lesions and is most likely to occur in infants;

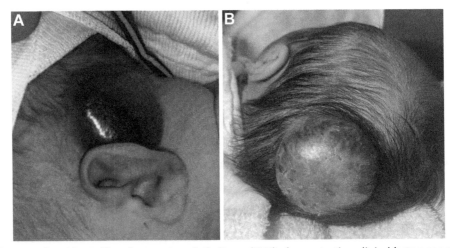

Fig. 4. Photographs of kaposiform hemangioendothelioma (KHE), demonstrating clinical heterogeneity. (*A*) Infant with solitary purpuric and tense tumor of the scalp. Coagulopathy was not present. (*B*) Infant with solitary vascular-appearing tumor of the scalp that was soft. Infant had severe thrombocytopenia and hypofibrinogenemia consistent with Kasabach–Merritt phenomenon (KMP).

however, the development of KMP in children and young adults has been reported.[52] Biopsy or excision of KHE in the setting of uncontrolled KMP, despite attempted correction of coagulopathy, is a risk for bleeding. Thus, biopsy may not be able to be performed safely.

Treatment of KHE is highly dependent on the presence of KMP. Without treatment, KHE with KMP is progressive and can lead to fatal hemorrhage, multiorgan failure, and death. If the lesion is amenable to resection, complete excision is preferred and considered curative. However, given its infiltrative nature, complete removal of the tumor is rarely possible, and if KMP is present, is at high risk for bleeding complications. Unlike other vascular anomalies, the molecular mechanism for KHE has not been convincingly identified to date. However, the discovery of sirolimus, a potent mTOR inhibitor, as an efficacious treatment for KHE with KMP suggests that the etiology causes disruptions of endothelial receptor intracellular signaling pathways such as PIK3CA/AKT or RAS/MAPK/MEK.[3] Before widespread sirolimus availability, a regimen of daily corticosteroids and weekly intravenous vincristine was used to treat KHE with KMP.[53] In the prospective phase 2 clinical trial on the safety and efficacy of sirolimus for the treatment of complicated vascular anomalies, Adams and colleagues reported excellent disease outcomes for patients with KHE and KMP.[54] Since then, vincristine use has substantially declined given the need for weekly infusions and central line access as well as the short- and long-term side-effects.[55] Today, the initial treatment of KHE with KMP most commonly consists of oral sirolimus and corticosteroid, with steroids typically weaning off over several months. Depending on the clinical severity, vincristine may also be added to this regimen . The medication regimen should be managed by a hematologist/oncologist familiar with these drugs and the necessary monitoring and dose adjustments.

Management of the hematologic abnormalities associated with KHE and KMP is another critical aspect of care. Maintenance of adequate hematologic parameters in individuals with KMP, particularly neonates, is important and ideally managed by a hematologist/oncologist with familiarity of KHE. Given platelet trapping and overactivation in the tumor, platelet transfusion should be avoided as this can not only worsen the coagulopathy but engorge the tumor and cause increased pain.[56] Generally, platelet transfusion is advised to only be given for active bleeding or immediately before or during a surgery with more than minimal risk of bleeding.[57] However, neonates and infants, particularly those born prematurely, do have specific platelet transfusion thresholds, generally determined by neonatally, given their physiology and risk of intracranial hemorrhage. Given risk of bleeding, fibrinogen is typically advised to be maintained more than 75 to 100 mg/dL (if not higher in neonates or premature infants) with either cryoprecipitate or fresh frozen plasma; a higher threshold should be considered in the presence of bleeding. Red blood cell transfusions do not negatively affect the tumor and can be given as needed for clinical reasons.[51,57]

Treatment of KHE without KMP depends on the presence of symptoms and/or complications such as pain or functional limitations that negatively impact the patient's quality of life.[53] If complete surgical excision is not possible or does not provide adequate improvement, physical therapy, orthopedic evaluation, and custom compression therapy are recommended. Oral sirolimus, as monotherapy, can also be considered with the aim of titrating to the lowest dose that alleviates pain and/or improves symptoms. Aspirin or other antiplatelet therapy can also be considered.[57]

CLINICS CARE POINTS

- Infantile hemangiomas are the most common tumor occurring in children.
- Oral propranolol is first-line treatment of complicated infantile hemangiomas.
- There are no effective drug therapies for congenital hemangiomas.
- Kasabach-Merritt phenomenon is only associated with Kaposiform Hemangioendothelioma and is life-threatening.

DISCLOSURE

The authors have no conflicts of interest to disclose.

REFERENCES

1. Léauté-Labrèze C, Dumas de la Roque E, Hubiche T, et al. Propranolol for severe hemangiomas of infancy. N Engl J Med 2008;358(24): 2649–51.
2. ISSVA Classification of vascular anomalies 2018, International Society for the Study of Vascular Anomalies. Available at "issva.org/classification" Accessed July 22, 2023. . https://www.issva.org/UserFiles/file/ISSVA-Classification-2018.pdf. Accessed June 2, 2020.

3. Hammill AM, Wentzel M, Gupta A, et al. Sirolimus for the treatment of complicated vascular anomalies in children. Pediatr Blood Cancer 2011;57(6):1018–24.

4. Krowchuk DP, Frieden IJ, Mancini AJ, et al. Clinical Practice Guideline for the Management of Infantile Hemangiomas. Pediatrics 2019;143(1).

5. Darrow DH, Greene AK, Mancini AJ, et al. Diagnosis and Management of Infantile Hemangioma. Pediatrics 2015;136(4):e1060–104.

6. Adams DM, Ricci KW. Infantile Hemangiomas in the Head and Neck Region. Otolaryngol Clin North Am 2018;51(1):77–87.

7. Greenberger S, Bischoff J. Pathogenesis of infantile haemangioma. Br J Dermatol 2013;169(1):12–9.

8. Hoeger PH, Harper JI, Baselga E, et al. Treatment of infantile haemangiomas: recommendations of a European expert group. Eur J Pediatr 2015;174(7):855–65.

9. van Vugt LJ, van der Vleuten CJM, Flucke U, et al. The utility of GLUT1 as a diagnostic marker in cutaneous vascular anomalies: A review of literature and recommendations for daily practice. Pathol Res Pract 2017;213(6):591–7.

10. Huang L, Nakayama H, Klagsbrun M, et al. Glucose transporter 1-positive endothelial cells in infantile hemangioma exhibit features of facultative stem cells. Stem Cell 2015;33(1):133–45.

11. Boscolo E, Bischoff J. Vasculogenesis in infantile hemangioma. Angiogenesis 2009;12(2):197–207.

12. Baselga E, Roe E, Coulie J, et al. Risk Factors for Degree and Type of Sequelae After Involution of Untreated Hemangiomas of Infancy. JAMA Dermatol 2016;152(11):1239–43.

13. Drolet BA, Frommelt PC, Chamlin SL, et al. Initiation and use of propranolol for infantile hemangioma: report of a consensus conference. Pediatrics 2013;131(1):128–40.

14. Léauté-Labrèze C, Hoeger P, Mazereeuw-Hautier J, et al. A randomized, controlled trial of oral propranolol in infantile hemangioma. N Engl J Med 2015;372(8):735–46.

15. Malik MA, Menon P, Rao KL, et al. Effect of propranolol vs prednisolone vs propranolol with prednisolone in the management of infantile hemangioma: a randomized controlled study. J Pediatr Surg 2013;48(12):2453–9.

16. Bauman NM, McCarter RJ, Guzzetta PC, et al. Propranolol vs prednisolone for symptomatic proliferating infantile hemangiomas: a randomized clinical trial. JAMA Otolaryngol Head Neck Surg 2014;140(4):323–30.

17. Pope E, Chakkittakandiyil A, Lara-Corrales I, et al. Expanding the therapeutic repertoire of infantile haemangiomas: cohort-blinded study of oral nadolol compared with propranolol. Br J Dermatol 2013;168(1):222–4.

18. Ji Y, Wang Q, Chen S, et al. Oral atenolol therapy for proliferating infantile hemangioma: A prospective study. Medicine (Baltim) 2016;95(24):e3908.

19. Bayart CB, Tamburro JE, Vidimos AT, et al. Atenolol Versus Propranolol for Treatment of Infantile Hemangiomas During the Proliferative Phase: A Retrospective Noninferiority Study. Pediatr Dermatol 2017;34(4):413–21.

20. Chakkittakandiyil A, Phillips R, Frieden IJ, et al. Timolol maleate 0.5% or 0.1% gel-forming solution for infantile hemangiomas: a retrospective, multicenter, cohort study. Pediatr Dermatol 2012;29(1):28–31.

21. Anwar F, Mahmood E, Sharif S, et al. Topical Application of 0.5% Timolol Maleate Hydrogel for the Treatment of Superficial Infantile Hemangiomas. J Drugs Dermatol 2023;22(6):594–8.

22. Zheng L, Li Y. Effect of topical timolol on response rate and adverse events in infantile hemangioma: a meta-analysis. Arch Dermatol Res 2018;310(4):261–9.

23. Novoa M, Baselga E, Beltran S, et al. Interventions for infantile haemangiomas of the skin. Cochrane Database Syst Rev 2018;4(4):Cd006545.

24. Frommelt P, Juern A, Siegel D, et al. Adverse Events in Young and Preterm Infants Receiving Topical Timolol for Infantile Hemangioma. Pediatr Dermatol 2016;33(4):405–14.

25. Greenberger S, Yuan S, Walsh LA, et al. Rapamycin suppresses self-renewal and vasculogenic potential of stem cells isolated from infantile hemangioma. J Invest Dermatol 2011;131(12):2467–76.

26. Kaylani S, Theos AJ, Pressey JG. Treatment of infantile hemangiomas with sirolimus in a patient with PHACE syndrome. Pediatr Dermatol 2013;30(6):e194–7.

27. Dávila-Osorio VL, Iznardo H, Roé E, et al. Propranolol-resistant infantile hemangioma successfully treated with sirolimus. Pediatr Dermatol 2020;37(4):684–6.

28. Xue L, Sun C, Xu DP, et al. Clinical Outcomes of Infants With Periorbital Hemangiomas Treated With Oral Propranolol. J Oral Maxillofac Surg 2016;74(11):2193–9.

29. Yuan SM, Cui L, Guo Y, et al. Management of periorbital hemangioma by intralesional glucocorticoids and systemic propranolol: a single-center retrospective study. Int J Clin Exp Med 2014;7(4):962–7.

30. Painter SL, Hildebrand GD. Topical timolol maleate 0.5% solution for the management of deep periocular infantile hemangiomas. J Aapos 2016;20(2):172–4.e171.

31. Elluru RG, Friess MR, Richter GT, et al. Multicenter Evaluation of the Effectiveness of Systemic Propranolol in the Treatment of Airway Hemangiomas. Otolaryngol Head Neck Surg 2015;153(3):452–60.

32. TJ OL, Messner A. Subglottic hemangioma. Otolaryngol Clin North Am 2008;41(5):903–11. viii-ix.

33. Metry DW, Garzon MC, Drolet BA, et al. PHACE syndrome: current knowledge, future directions. Pediatr Dermatol 2009;26(4):381–98.

34. Metry D, Heyer G, Hess C, et al. Consensus Statement on Diagnostic Criteria for PHACE Syndrome. Pediatrics 2009;124(5):1447–56.

35. Garzon MC, Epstein LG, Heyer GL, et al. PHACE Syndrome: Consensus-Derived Diagnosis and Care Recommendations. J Pediatr 2016;178:24–33.e22.

36. Baselga E, Cordisco MR, Garzon M, et al. Rapidly involuting congenital haemangioma associated with transient thrombocytopenia and coagulopathy: a case series. Br J Dermatol 2008;158(6):1363–70.

37. Liang MG, Frieden IJ. Infantile and congenital hemangiomas. Semin Pediatr Surg 2014;23(4):162–7.

38. North PE. Pediatric Vascular Tumors and Malformations. Surgical Pathology Clinics 2010;3(3):455–94.

39. Olsen GM, Nackers A, Drolet BA. Infantile and congenital hemangiomas. Semin Pediatr Surg 2020;29(5):150969.

40. Giblin AV, Clover AJ, Athanassopoulos A, et al. Pyogenic granuloma - the quest for optimum treatment: audit of treatment of 408 cases. J Plast Reconstr Aesthetic Surg 2007;60(9):1030–5.

41. Wollina U, Langner D, França K, et al. Pyogenic Granuloma - A Common Benign Vascular Tumor with Variable Clinical Presentation: New Findings and Treatment Options. Open Access Maced J Med Sci 2017;5(4):423–6.

42. Wine Lee L, Goff KL, Lam JM, et al. Treatment of pediatric pyogenic granulomas using β-adrenergic receptor antagonists. Pediatr Dermatol 2014;31(2):203–7.

43. Piraccini BM, Alessandrini A, Dika E, et al. Topical propranolol 1% cream for pyogenic granulomas of the nail: open-label study in 10 patients. J Eur Acad Dermatol Venereol 2016;30(5):901–2.

44. Oke I, Alkharashi M, Petersen RA, et al. Treatment of Ocular Pyogenic Granuloma With Topical Timolol. JAMA Ophthalmol 2017;135(4):383–5.

45. Queisser A, Seront E, Boon LM, et al. Genetic Basis and Therapies for Vascular Anomalies. Circ Res 2021;129(1):155–73.

46. Zukerberg LR, Nickoloff BJ, Weiss SW. Kaposiform hemangioendothelioma of infancy and childhood. An aggressive neoplasm associated with Kasabach-Merritt syndrome and lymphangiomatosis. Am J Surg Pathol 1993;17(4):321–8.

47. Croteau SE, Liang MG, Kozakewich HP, et al. Kaposiform hemangioendothelioma: atypical features and risks of Kasabach-Merritt phenomenon in 107 referrals. J Pediatr 2013;162(1):142–7.

48. Croteau SE, Kozakewich HP, Perez-Atayde AR, et al. Kaposiform lymphangiomatosis: a distinct aggressive lymphatic anomaly. J Pediatr 2014;164(2):383–8.

49. Foley LS, Kulungowski AM. Vascular Anomalies in Pediatrics. Adv Pediatr 2015;62(1):227–55.

50. Szabo SNP. Histopathology and pathogenesis of vascular tumors and malformations. In: North PEST, editor. Vascular tumors and developmental malformations: Pathogenic mechanisms and molecular diagnosis. NY: New York Springer; 2016. p. 1–62.

51. Ricci KW, Brandão LR. Coagulation issues in vascular anomalies. Semin Pediatr Surg 2020;29(5):150966.

52. O'Rafferty C, O'Regan GM, Irvine AD, et al. Recent advances in the pathobiology and management of Kasabach-Merritt phenomenon. Br J Haematol 2015;171(1):38–51.

53. Drolet BA, Trenor CC 3rd, Brandao LR, et al. Consensus-derived practice standards plan for complicated Kaposiform hemangioendothelioma. J Pediatr 2013;163(1):285–91.

54. Adams DM, Trenor CC 3rd, Hammill AM, et al. Efficacy and Safety of Sirolimus in the Treatment of Complicated Vascular Anomalies. Pediatrics 2016;137(2):e20153257.

55. Ricci KW. Advances in the Medical Management of Vascular Anomalies. Semin Intervent Radiol 2017;34(3):239–49.

56. Phillips WG, Marsden JR. Kasabach-Merritt syndrome exacerbated by platelet transfusion. J R Soc Med 1993;86(4):231–2.

57. Nakano TAFI. Kaposiform Hemangioendothelioma and Kasabach-Merritt Phenomenon: Management of Coagulopathy and Treatment Options. In: Trenor II CCAD, editor. Vascular anomalies. Switzerland: Springer; 2020. p. 63–88.

Medical Management and Therapeutic Updates on Vascular Anomalies of the Head and Neck: Part 2

Jorie Gatts, MD[a,1], Srinivasa R. Chandra, BDS, MD, FDS, FIBCSOMS[b,*], Kiersten Ricci, MD[c,d,1]

KEYWORDS

- Hemangioma • Vascular malformation • Propranolol • Timolol • Sirolimus • Alpelisib • Trametinib
- Bevacizumab

KEY POINTS

- First-line treatment of complicated infantile hemangiomas is with beta-adrenergic antagonist, oral propranolol. Topical timolol can be considered for less complicated superficial infantile hemangiomas.
- Kaposiform hemangioendothelioma is a locally aggressive vascular tumor that is associated with a life-threatening coagulopathy, Kasabach-Merritt phenomenon. Early consultation with hematology/oncology for management is critical.
- Sirolimus, a potent mTOR inhibitor, has been demonstrated to be a safe and efficacious treatment for complicated vascular anomalies.
- Currently, most molecular and targeted therapies, other than alpeselib, are currently used off-label and on a compassionate basis for vascular anomaly management.
- Surgical management can be an adjunct to medical therapy for symptom management of vascular anomalies.

INTRODUCTION

Vascular anomalies (VAs), broadly classified as non-malignant tumors and malformations, consist of a multitude of disorders that have a wide range of symptoms and complications as well as overlapping clinical, radiologic, and histologic findings. Although usually difficult, distinguishing between non-malignant vascular tumors and malformations, as well as the precise diagnosis within these distinctions, is critical because prognosis, therapy, and chronicity of care vary greatly. VAs in the head and neck area are common, associated with high morbidity, and can be life-threatening. Potential complications of head/neck VA include airway obstruction, vision and hearing impairment, facial disfigurement, infection, thromboembolic events, coagulopathy with bleeding, feeding and speech issues as well as psychosocial and economic stressors.

Optimal management of complex VAs aims to not only treat acute issues, such as infection or

[a] Department of Pediatrics, University of Cincinnati College of Medicine, Cincinnati, OH, USA; [b] Department of Oral and Maxillofacial Surgery, Oregon Health and Sciences University, Portland, OR, USA; [c] Hemangioma and Vascular Malformation Center, Cancer and Blood Diseases Institute, Cincinnati Children's Hospital Medical Center, Cincinnati, OH 45229, USA; [d] Division of Hematology, Cancer and Blood Diseases Institute, Cincinnati Children's Hospital Medical Center, 3333 Burnet Avenue, MLC 7015, Cincinnati, OH 45229, USA
[1] Both authors contributed equally.
* Corresponding author. Oral and Maxillofacial- Head and Neck Oncology and Microvascular Surgery, Oregon Health & Science University, 3181 SW Sam Jackson Park Rd, Portland, OR 97239.
E-mail address: chandrsr@ohsu.edu

Oral Maxillofacial Surg Clin N Am 36 (2024) 115–123
https://doi.org/10.1016/j.coms.2023.09.012
1042-3699/24/© 2023 Elsevier Inc. All rights reserved.

effusion, but also prevent potential future complications and improve physical functioning and quality of life. Historically, medical treatment for VAs focused on managing complications with pain control, antibiotics, dental hygiene, and compression garments, which are often uncomfortable and impractical in the head and neck area.

In addition to the development of a formal VA classification system, adopted by the International Society for the Study of Vascular Anomalies (ISSVA), the serendipitous discovery of sirolimus, a mammalian target of rapamycin inhibitor, as an efficacious treatment for complicated VA, boosted interest in the field, propelled clinical and basic science research, and began to shift the treatment approach.[1,2] Similarly, the discovery of the efficaciousness of beta-adrenergic blockage, specifically with oral propranolol, revolutionized the treatment paradigm for infantile hemangiomas.[3] Oral propranolol quickly became first-line therapy and substantially lessened the need for interventions like surgical excision and laser therapy.

Study of the pathophysiology and molecular biology of vascular tumors and malformations has rapidly expanded. In the last decade, germline, and somatic mutations in the endothelial receptor intracellular signaling pathways, phosphatidylinositol-4,5-bisphosphate 3-kinase (PIK3)/AKT and RAS (rat sarcoma)/mitogen activated protein kinase (MAPK)/MAPK kinase(MEK), have been identified in numerous VA.[4–6] While optimal management of patients with complex VAs requires an interdisciplinary approach, these genomic discoveries have led to new therapeutic options and an increasing importance of the hematologist/oncologist within multidisciplinary VA care teams. This article discusses the medical management for non-malignant vascular tumors, vascular malformations, and latest drug therapies.

VASCULAR MALFORMATIONS

VAs vary with phenotypic expression. The abnormalities may also be a minor or major component of the phenotype of a syndrome such as PIK3 catalytic subunit alpha (PIK3CA)-related overgrowth spectrum (PROS) and capillary-lymphatic-venous malformation in Klippel-Trenaunay syndrome (KTS) or CLOVES (congenital, lipomatous, overgrowth, vascular malformation, epidermal nevi, spinal anomalies) (Access of complete ISSVA classification at: www.issva.org/classification). Vascular malformations are described as either slow flow or fast flow, depending on the presence or absence of an arterial component. This differentiation is important because high-flow lesions have unique complications (eg, high-output cardiac failure), and

management has been primarily surgical due to the ineffectiveness of sirolimus, the only previously known targeted medication for VA.

Recent advancements in genetic testing have allowed for the identification of germline and somatic mutations that disrupt endothelial receptor intracellular signaling pathways, such as PIK3/AKT and RAS/MAPK, resulting in correlation of phenotype and genotype in VAs.[4–6] PIK3/AKT or RAS/MAPK pathway overactivation results in dysregulation of normal cellular functions, leading to cellular growth, survival advantage, and angiogenesis, which is believed to be the driving force for the development and/or progression of VA. As a result of a greater understanding of the molecular pathophysiology of VA, disease-modifying drugs, originally created for malignancy, are now being used to target the altered cellular signaling pathways in VA. Except for alpelisib, recently Food and Drug Administration-approved for treatment of PROS, all molecularly targeted medications, including sirolimus, are currently used off-label. **Table 1** lists the known associated genetic mutation(s) for the VA phenotype. **Fig. 1** illustrates the molecular targets of medications used in vascular malformations.

Lymphatic Malformations

Lymphatic malformations (LMs) are slow-flow vascular malformations, composed of dilated lymphatic channels or cysts lined by lymphatic endothelial cells, associated with somatic *PIK3CA* activating mutations. Depending on the size of the fluid-filled cysts, LM are categorized as microcystic, macrocystic, or mixed. LMs are frequently noted at birth as soft, compressible lesions, with or without overlying skin discoloration; however, a small or deep lesion may not become apparent until it enlarges to produce symptoms or deformity. Superficial LM may produce cutaneous vesicles filled with lymphatic fluid and/or blood called lymphatic blebs. Large LM may also be diagnosed on prenatal imaging. Two-thirds of LMs occur in the head and neck area, some of which extend into the mediastinum, and may impede on the airway, resulting in life-threatening complications such as airway obstruction or tracheal deviation (**Fig. 2**).[7,8] Most LM are solitary or regional but can be diffuse or multifocal. LM is also associated with PROS including KTS and CLOVES, all of which are also associated with somatic *PIK3CA* mutations.

Acute enlargement is common and is typically caused by infection, inflammation, trauma, or intralesional bleeding. Intralesional hemorrhage can occur in the absence of injury. LMs have increased

Table 1
Identified gene mutations by phenotype of associated vascular anomaly

Diagnosis/Phenotype	Genetic Mutations
Lymphatic malformation, sporadic	PIK3CA
Klippel-Trenaunay syndrome (capillary-lymphatic-venous malformation [CLVM] or congenital venous malformation [CVM] with overgrowth of affected extremity)	PIK3CA
Congenital, lipomatous, overgrowth, vascular malformation, epidermal nevi, spinal anomalies (CLOVES) syndrome	PIK3CA
Megalencephaly-Capillary Malformation (MCM) or Megalencephaly-Capillary malformation-Polymicrogyria syndrome (MCAP)	PIK3CA
Generalized lymphatic anomaly (GLA)	PIK3CA
Kaposiform lymphangiomatosis (KLA)	NRAS
Venous malformations, sporadic	PIK3CA, TIE2/TEK
Glomuvenous malformation	GLMN
Multiple cutaneous and mucosal venous malformation (VMCM)	TIE2/TEK
Blue Rubber Bleb Nevus Syndrome (BRBNS)	TIE2/TEK
Arteriovenous malformations, extracranial and sporadic	MAP2K1, KRAS, NRAS, BRAF
Arteriovenous malformation, intracranial and sporadic	KRAS, BRAF
PTEN (phosphatase and tensin homolog) hamartoma	PTEN
Fibroadipose vascular anomaly	PIK3CA
Vein of Galen aneurysmal malformation, subtype of cerebral arteriovenous malformation (AVM)	EPHB4
Capillary Malformation-Arteriovenous Malformation Type 1 (CM-AVM1)	RASA1
Capillary Malformation-Arteriovenous Malformation Type 2 (CM-AVM2)	EPHB4
Hereditary Hemorrhagic Telangiectasia syndrome (HHT)	ACVRL1, ENG, SMAD4, GDF2/BMP9
Capillary Malformation, sporadic	GNAQ, GNA11
Sturge-Weber syndrome	GNAQ
Facial infiltrating lipomatosis	PIK3CA

risk for cellulitis or soft tissue infection, particularly if the LM involves the oral or nasal mucosa or lymphatic blebs are present. Antibiotics should be used to treat suspected bacterial infections, while non-steroidal anti-inflammatories or corticosteroids can be used to alleviate acute pain and/or substantial enlargement. Chronic issues such as pain, functional limitations, asymmetry, recurrent infection, or hemorrhage should be managed on an individualized basis. Treatment options include sclerotherapy, surgery, and disease-modifying medications such as sirolimus and alpelisib that both target the PIK3-AKT pathway.

Complex Lymphatic Anomalies

Complex lymphatic anomalies (CLAs) are rare, progressive diseases involving multifocal LM that are associated with high morbidity. CLA includes Gorham-Stout disease (GSD), generalized lymphatic anomaly (GLA), and kaposiform lymphangiomatosis (KLA). These diseases typically involve viscera and bone, in addition to the soft tissues and body cavities like isolated LM. Individuals can suffer from numerous complications such as lytic bone lesions, pleural and pericardial effusion, ascites, serious infection, coagulopathy, bleeding, and protein losses.[8] These conditions have phenotypic heterogeneity as well as overlapping symptoms, imaging features, and complications, making diagnosis challenging. However, there are clinical manifestations, radiologic findings, and genetic mutations that can differentiate these conditions. While GSD, GLA, and KLA all have bone involvement, only osteolytic lesions of GSD cause bone cortex destruction and frank loss of bone; GSD has a propensity to affect the calvarium, skull base, vertebrae, and bones of

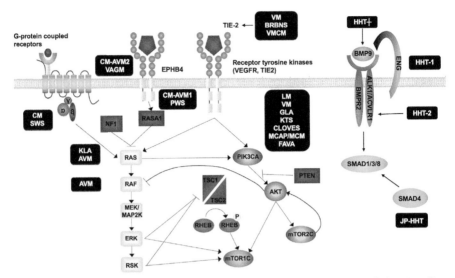

Fig. 1. Genetic alterations associated with vascular malformations in the major cellular signaling pathways. Abbreviations: AVM, arteriovenous malformation; BRBNS, Blue Rubber Bleb Nevus Syndrome; CM, capillary malformation; CM-AVM1, capillary malformation-arteriovenous malformation type 1; CM-AVM2, capillary malformation-arteriovenous malformation type 2; CLOVES, Congenital Lipomatous Overgrowth Vascular malformation Epidermal nevus Spinal anomalies syndrome; FAVA, fibroadipose vascular anomaly; GLA, generalized lymphatic anomaly; HHT†, HHT-like syndrome; HHT-1, hereditary hemorrhagic telangiectasia type 1; HHT-2, hereditary hemorrhagic telangiectasia type 2; JP-HHT, juvenile polyposis and hereditary hemorrhagic telangiectasia; KLA, kaposiform lymphangiomatosis; LM, lymphatic malformation; MCAP, megalencephaly-capillary malformation-polymicrogyria; MCM, megalencephaly-capillary malformation syndrome; PWS, Parkes-Weber syndrome; SWS, Sturge-Weber syndrome; VAGM, vein of Galen aneurysmal malformation; VM, venous malformation; VMCM, multiple cutaneous and mucosal venous malformation.

the upper body including the clavicle, sternum, and scapula.[9] KLA is the only CLA associated with coagulopathy, which is characterized by severe thrombocytopenia, hypofibrinogenemia, and bleeding propensity including hemorrhagic effusions. *PIK3CA* mutations have been discovered in GLA; in contrast, *RAS* mutations have been found in KLA. Casitas B lineage lymphoma gene mutation has also been found in KLA, which is within the RAS/MAPK pathway.[10] The genetic mutation in GSD has not yet been identified. Given the diffuse nature and significant morbidity of CLA,

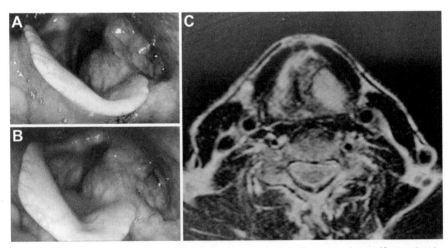

Fig. 2. Endoscopy photographs and MRI imaging of a patient with slow-flow vascular malformation involving the airway. (*A*) Endoscopy images of the left laryngeal area and (*B*) piriform fossa. (*C*) Magnetic resonance imaging, axial view, of the same patient demonstrating intense contrast uptake with left vocal cord deviation in the laryngeal area.

systemic medical therapeutics play an important role not only in the treatment of clinical manifestations but also in the prevention of progression. Bisphosphonates such as zoledronic acid are also frequently used when lytic bone lesions are present. Correct diagnosis of CLA is critical because use of a targeted drug in the opposing pathway could potentially worsen the disease. Potential molecularly targeted drugs for CLA include sirolimus, alpelisib, and MEK inhibitors.

Venous Malformations

Venous malformations (VMs) are slow-flow vascular malformations composed of ectatic, dysmorphic venous vessels that may be solitary/isolated, regional, multifocal (separate malformations involving multiple body areas), or extensive (involving multiple body regions or entire extremities). Like LM, VMs are also associated with PROS, KTS, and CLOVES. Superficial VMs appear as abnormal veins or blue-purple skin discoloration, while deeper VMs may only be palpable as a soft tissue swelling or may not be detectable on examination if within muscle or bone. VM typically increases in volume with increased venous pressure (eg, Valsalva maneuver or straining), when the affected body area is dependent, or with exercise.[11] VM may also occur in the aerodigestive tract, potentially causing airway compromise, dysphagia, and gastrointestinal (GI) bleeding.[11] Although VM can occur anywhere in the body, 40% occur in the head and neck, most commonly in the muscles of mastication, the lip, and the tongue.[12–14]

Due to the abnormally decreased or stagnant blood flow through the distorted vessels, affected individuals are at increased risk for thrombophlebitis and thrombosis of the VM.[15] Individuals are also predisposed to phleboliths, which are organized thrombi that have calcified. Risk for deep vein thrombosis and venous thromboembolism is highly dependent on an individual's malformation and connections to the normal deep venous system. During periods of systemic inflammation, local injury, or hormone fluctuations, VM can develop thrombophlebitis and become more painful and swollen. In pubertal females, progestin-only hormonal control or oral contraceptives are recommended given the known increased risk of thrombosis with estrogen-containing medications in addition to the high likelihood of clinical worsening of the VM. Anticoagulation with low molecular weight heparin or direct-acting oral anticoagulants, such as rivaroxaban or apixaban, should be considered for patients with recurrent thrombophlebitis at prophylactic or treatment dosing. Aspirin and clopidogrel have been reportedly used, albeit with less success, and caution should be used as these drugs also should be stopped 5 to 7 days prior to a procedure to avoid bleeding complications.

Affected individuals, particularly those with extensive or multifocal venous involvement, frequently have an elevated D-dimer, suggesting an increased generation of thrombin, accompanied by fibrinolysis, presumably due to recurrent thrombophlebitis and/or chronic formation of microthrombi.[15] Elevated D-dimer and concurrent moderate to severe hypofibrinogenemia occur in approximately 6% to 10% of patients.[16] Despite hypofibrinogenemia and/or thrombocytopenia, individuals do not appear to have increased bleeding without an additional inciting factor.[15] Both venous thromboembolism and worsening coagulopathy have occurred, speculatively due to manipulation or trauma of the malformation with surgery, sclerotherapy, embolization, or injury.[17–19] Sirolimus has been reported to improve thrombophlebitis, phlebolith formation, and laboratory hematologic abnormalities in patients with VMs or combined VMs.[20] If hematologic abnormalities are present and surgical intervention is planned, pre-operative hematology/oncology consultation is highly advised.

Venous malformations are caused by both inherited and somatic mutations. Germline VMs include glomuvenous malformation, inherited by a loss-of-function *GLMN* mutation, and multiple cutaneous and mucosal VM syndromes, inherited by autosomal dominant activating mutations in *TEK/TIE2*. Lacking family history, blue rubber bleb syndrome is another multifocal VM that is associated with somatic *TEK/TIE2* mutations but has a propensity to involve the aerodigestive tract and cause GI bleeding. Sporadically occurring VMs are associated with either somatic *PIK3CA* or *TEK/TIE2* mutations. While the phase 2 clinical trial of sirolimus treatment did not include isolated VM, the results suggested improvements in complicated malformations with a venous component.[21] Additional studies and case series have provided additional support for the benefits of sirolimus treatment in VM.[9,22–25] Prospective clinical trials for use of molecularly targeted drugs in simple/isolated VM are lacking. In clinical practice, sirolimus may alleviate symptoms and provide clinical benefits for VM. The PIK3CA inhibitor, alpelisib, may also be beneficial in VM with a *PIK3CA* mutation.

Arteriovenous Malformations

Arteriovenous malformations (AVMs) are high-flow or fast-flow malformations caused by aberrant development of vasculature that abnormally connects arteries and veins, disrupting blood flow and oxygen circulation. Since these 2 types of vessels are normally connected by high-resistance capillary beds, venous vessel walls are not intended to handle the high-pressure blood flow occurring in AVM. As a result, the venous component of the AVM becomes permanently altered and weak, making these vessels vulnerable to bleeding and rupture. AVM can occur anywhere in the body and typically progress over time. The arterial to venous shunting leads to ischemia with destruction of surrounding tissue, pain, ulceration, bleeding, and potentially cardiac overload. AVMs have traditionally been thought to be congenital, arising from dysfunction of developmental pathways implicated in vasculogenesis and/or vascular maturation. However, de novo AVM formation has been described in the brain and extra-cranially.[26]

Treatment of AVM has been mostly surgical and is challenging with embolization or resection frequently resulting in subsequent recurrence or expansion of collateral vessels in up to 80% of cases. Additionally, incomplete resection and embolization can cause aggressive growth of the remaining nidus (where feeding arteries link directly to draining veins), and the risk of progression is up to 50% during the first 5 years, with recurrences possible 10 years later.[27] Embolization materials (coils, ethanol, cyanoacrylate, polyvinyl alcohol known as Onyx, fibrin glue, etc.) have varying rates of successful AVM regression and differing complications.

Extracranial AVM most commonly affect the head and neck area (47.4%), with an estimated 50% of head and neck AVM affecting the oral and maxillofacial region.[27] Bleeding complications are common for individuals with angiodysplasias or AVM involving mucosal surfaces, particularly in the nasopharyngeal and GI tracts, and cause significant morbidity. Supportive care with blood product transfusion and intravenous iron replacement is critical but is only supportive and disruptive to affected patients' lives. Surgical interventions can be beneficial but may be limited or insufficient due to the diffuse nature of these vascular diseases. As a result, there is an increased interest in using angiogenesis inhibitors, many of which are now employed in cancer treatment regimens, to treat these problematic vascular lesions complicated by bleeding. In sporadically occurring extracranial AVM, activating mutations in *MAP2K1*, *KRAS*, *NRAS*, and *BRAF* have been identified.[28] El Sissy and colleagues reported that *KRAS* mutations were associated with severe extended facial AVM, for which relapse after surgical resection is frequently

observed, while *MAP2K1* variants were associated with less severe AVM located on the lips.[29] All identified mutations in sporadically occurring AVM are within the RAS/MAPK pathway, suggesting that MEK inhibitors may be potential therapeutic agents for individuals with extracranial AVM. In 2 case reports, children with problematic AVM were treated off-label with oral trametinib and reported decreased blood flow through the AVM as well as reduced vessel caliber after 6 months of therapy.[30,31]

Intracranial AVM can lead to significant neurologic disability or death, usually because of intracranial hemorrhage (ICH).[32,33] Over half of brain AVM detected will first present with hemorrhage, and previous hemorrhage is the most important indicator for subsequent bleeding.[34,35] In the absence of ICH, persistent headache is the most common symptom. Intracerebral AVM are high-flow lesions and distinctly different from cavernous malformations of the brain, which are low flow. Approximately 95% of brain AVMs are sporadic while the remainder are associated with hereditary conditions of which hereditary hemorrhagic telangiectasia (HHT) is the most common.[36] In sporadic brain AVM, *KRAS* mutations have been recently identified in most patients, and more rarely *BRAF* mutations.[26] *EPHB4* mutations have also been found in sporadic vein of Galen aneurysmal malformations, which are a subtype of cerebral AVM.[28] Pathogenesis of sporadic intracranial AVM is not understood, but well-known associated factors such as angiogenic factors and inflammatory cytokines likely influence the development of brain AVM.[36] Inhibiting the RAS/MAPK cascade with MEK inhibition may be a promising approach to treating non-hereditary brain AVM.

Capillary malformation-AVM (CM-AVM) syndrome is an inherited autosomal dominant disorder with high penetrance characterized by multiple cutaneous CM and risk of having 1 or more AVM and/or arteriovenous fistulas. CM-AVM is subdivided by its causative mutations,RAS P21 protein activator 1 (*RASA1*) and ephrin-type B receptor 4 (*EPHB4*), into CM-AVM1 and CM-AVM2, respectively.[37] CM-AVM1 is caused by a heterozygous loss-of-function mutation in the *RASA1*, which encodes RASp21, a protein that acts as a suppressor of RAS function. CM-AVM2 is caused by a loss-of-function mutation in EPHB4, which, along with its ligand Ephrin B2, plays a significant role in arteriovenous differentiation.[28] Of note, Parkes-Weber syndrome is a phenotype that is characterized by CM-AVM and hypertrophy of the underlying bone and tissue, resulting in limb overgrowth. Since Parkes-Weber syndrome is a phenotype, the associated *RASA1* mutation may be germline or somatic. Molecularly targeted medications have not been widely used to treat CM-AVM patients yet, but case reports and small series are emerging.

HHT is an inherited autosomal dominant disease, with an estimated prevalence of 1 in 5000, which is characterized by AVM that can occur in the brain, lungs, liver, and spine and mucocutaneous telangiectasias.[38] Diagnosis is based on the Curacao criteria, published by Shovlin and colleagues in 2000 and revised in 2020.[39,40] Clinical symptoms vary not only among HHT patients but even within families carrying the same disease-causing mutation. The most common symptom is recurrent, spontaneous epistaxis because of telangiectatic lesions in the nasal mucosa, affecting 95% of HHT patients, followed by GI bleeding occurring in 13% to 30% of affected individuals.[41] Severity of epistaxis and GI bleeding can range from occasional and brief to life-threatening and lead to red blood cell transfusion and intravenous iron infusion-dependence.[42] With age, the amount of telangiectasias increases, and epistaxis and/or GI bleeds typically worsen, leading to iron deficiency anemia, poorer quality of life, and increased healthcare resource utilization, including the need for frequent transfusions and hospitalizations. Treatment of epistaxis can range from topical intranasal medications to laser, nasal packing, and nasal closure in the very severe.[43] Telangiectatic lesions in the GI tract are addressed with thermal probes or local laser treatment.

AVM can form in the brain in up to 10% of HHT patients, the lungs in 15% to 45%, and the liver in 75% of patients. Chronic bleeding or acute rupture of these AVM can result in severe or potentially fatal complications, including internal hemorrhage, embolic or hemorrhagic stroke, seizures, migraines, brain abscesses, high-output cardiac failure, and pulmonary hypertension.[43,44]

In 97% of patients with a definite clinical diagnosis of HHT, a causative loss-of-function mutation is identified in 1 of 3 genes: endoglin (ENG), activin receptor-like kinase-1, and mothers against decapentaplegic homolog 4 (SMAD4).[45] Recently, Balachandar and colleagues proposed that a heterozygous GDF2/BMP9 variant is also a cause of HHT associated with pulmonary AVM.[46] Researchers are beginning to make strides in correlating genotype-phenotype, with the ENG mutation more frequently associated with the presence of pulmonary AVM and brain vascular malformations whereas GI bleeding was more often associated with SMAD4 genotype.[44] Each of these 3 genes encodes proteins involved in the TGF/BMP superfamily signaling pathways and plays an important role in angiogenic balance, making vascular endothelial growth factor an appealing target for molecular-based drug therapy. Use of anti-angiogenic drugs for problematic HHT-associated bleeding is addressed later in this article.

Capillary Malformations

Capillary malformations (CM), previously referred to as "port wine stains" or PWS, consist of abnormally dilated capillaries within the skin and mucosa, appearing as pink to red macules that blanch with pressure. When involving the face, CM may thicken and darken over time and develop inflammatory nodules or overlying pyogenic granulomas. In CM that has high blood flow, soft tissue and/or bony overgrowth may also occur. Identified gene mutations in CM include GNAQ and GNA11.[47] Due to phenotypic heterogeneity and variable penetrance, some individuals with a family history of HHT or CM-AVM may present with CM only. If a patient has CM only but tests positive for germline mutation consistent with HHT or CM-AVM, then the individual needs referral to a specialty vascular center for further comprehensive evaluation including family history/assessment.

The indications and effectiveness of molecularly targeted medications remain unclear for CM. Unsurprisingly, given the different causal mechanisms of these conditions, systemic and topical sirolimus have not demonstrated any benefits for CM or the capillary components of combined malformations.[21,48,49] In fact, combined use of topical sirolimus and pulsed dye laser for treatment of CM may result in increased complications such as delayed ulceration and increased systemic absorption. Topical MEK inhibition could potentially be a therapeutic option in the future for inflammatory issues related to CM. Sturge-Weber syndrome, arising from a somatic GNAQ mutation, is a congenital neurologic disorder that is associated with a CM on the face, with high-risk areas including the upper eyelid area, forehead, and scalp. One small prospective study investigated use of sirolimus in children with Sturge-Weber syndrome and suggested that sirolimus may be beneficial for cognitive impairments, such as in those with impaired processing speed or a history of stroke-like episodes.[50]

Continued as Part 3 of 3 parts in the following article.

DISCLOSURE

The authors have no conflict of interest to disclose.

REFERENCES

1. ISSVA Classification of vascular anomalies 2018, International Society for the Study of Vascular Anomalies. Available at "issva.org/classification" Accessed July 22, 2023. https://www.issva.org/UserFiles/file/ISSVA-Classification-2018.pdf. Accessed June 2, 2020.

2. Hammill AM, Wentzel M, Gupta A, et al. Sirolimus for the treatment of complicated vascular anomalies in children. Pediatr Blood Cancer 2011;57(6):1018–24.

3. Léauté-Labrèze C, Dumas de la Roque E, Hubiche T, et al. Propranolol for severe hemangiomas of infancy. N Engl J Med 2008;358(24):2649–51.

4. Greene AK, Goss JA. Vascular anomalies: From a clinicohistologic to a genetic framework. Plast Reconstr Surg 2018;141(5):709e–17e.

5. Wassef M, Blei F, Adams D, et al. Vascular anomalies classification: recommendations from the international society for the study of vascular anomalies. Pediatrics 2015;136(1):e203–14.

6. Queisser A, Seront E, Boon LM, et al. Genetic basis and therapies for vascular anomalies. Circ Res 2021;129(1):155–73.

7. Krowchuk DP, Frieden IJ, Mancini AJ, et al. Clinical practice guideline for the management of infantile hemangiomas. Pediatrics 2019;143(1).

8. Ricci KW, Iacobas I. How we approach the diagnosis and management of complex lymphatic anomalies. Pediatr Blood Cancer 2022;69(Suppl 3):e28985.

9. Ricci KW, Hammill AM, Mobberley-Schuman P, et al. Efficacy of systemic sirolimus in the treatment of generalized lymphatic anomaly and Gorham-Stout disease. Pediatr Blood Cancer 2019;66(5):e27614.

10. Foster JB, Li D, March ME, et al. Kaposiform lymphangiomatosis effectively treated with MEK inhibition. EMBO Mol Med 2020;12(10):e12324.

11. Gallant SC, Chewning RH, Orbach DB, et al. Contemporary Management of Vascular Anomalies of the Head and Neck-Part 1: Vascular Malformations: A Review. JAMA Otolaryngol Head Neck Surg 2021;147(2):197–206.

12. Park H, Kim JS, Park H, et al. Venous malformations of the head and neck: A retrospective review of 82 cases. Arch Plast Surg 2019;46(1):23–33.

13. Richter GT, Braswell L. Management of venous malformations. Facial Plast Surg 2012;28(6):603–10.

14. Vogel SA, Hess CP, Dowd CF, et al. Early versus later presentations of venous malformations: where and why? Pediatr Dermatol 2013;30(5):534–40.

15. Ricci KW, Brandão LR. Coagulation issues in vascular anomalies. Semin Pediatr Surg 2020;29(5):150966.

16. Dompmartin A, Acher A, Thibon P, et al. Association of localized intravascular coagulopathy with venous malformations. Arch Dermatol 2008;144(7):873–7.

17. Adams DM. Special considerations in vascular anomalies: hematologic management. Clin Plast Surg 2011;38(1):153–60.

18. Mazoyer E, Enjolras O, Laurian C, et al. Coagulation abnormalities associated with extensive venous malformations of the limbs: differentiation from Kasabach-Merritt syndrome. Clin Lab Haematol 2002;24(4):243–51.

19. Mazoyer E, Enjolras O, Bisdorff A, et al. Coagulation disorders in patients with venous malformation of the limbs and trunk: a case series of 118 patients. Arch Dermatol 2008;144(7):861–7.

20. Mack JM, Verkamp B, Richter GT, et al. Effect of sirolimus on coagulopathy of slow-flow vascular malformations. Pediatr Blood Cancer 2019;66(10):e27896.

21. Adams DM, Trenor CC 3rd, Hammill AM, et al. Efficacy and Safety of Sirolimus in the Treatment of Complicated Vascular Anomalies. Pediatrics 2016;137(2). e20153257.

22. Engel ER, Hammill A, Adams D, et al. Response to sirolimus in capillary lymphatic venous malformations and associated syndromes: Impact on symptomatology, quality of life, and radiographic response. Pediatr Blood Cancer 2023;70(4):e30215.

23. Zhang G, Chen H, Zhen Z, et al. Sirolimus for treatment of verrucous venous malformation: A retrospective cohort study. J Am Acad Dermatol 2019;80(2):556–8.

24. Hammer J, Seront E, Duez S, et al. Sirolimus is efficacious in treatment for extensive and/or complex slow-flow vascular malformations: a monocentric prospective phase II study. Orphanet J Rare Dis 2018;13(1):191.

25. Maruani A, Tavernier E, Boccara O, et al. Sirolimus (Rapamycin) for Slow-Flow Malformations in Children: The Observational-Phase Randomized Clinical PERFORMUS Trial. JAMA Dermatol 2021;157(11):1289–98.

26. Vetiska S, Wälchli T, Radovanovic I, et al. Molecular and genetic mechanisms in brain arteriovenous malformations: new insights and future perspectives. Neurosurg Rev 2022;45(6):3573–93.

27. Fernández-Alvarez V, Suárez C, de Bree R, et al. Management of extracranial arteriovenous malformations of the head and neck. Auris Nasus Larynx 2020;47(2):181–90.

28. Nguyen HBL, Vikkula M. The Genetic Basis of Vascular Anomalies. In: vascular anomalies. Switzerland: Springer; 2020. p. 17–29. Trenor II CC AD.

29. El Sissy FN, Wassef M, Faucon B, et al. Somatic mutational landscape of extracranial arteriovenous malformations and phenotypic correlations. J Eur Acad Dermatol Venereol 2022;36(6):905–12.

30. Edwards EA, Phelps AS, Cooke D, et al. Monitoring Arteriovenous Malformation Response to Genotype-Targeted Therapy. Pediatrics 2020;146(3).

31. Lekwuttikarn R, Lim YH, Admani S, et al. Genotype-guided medical treatment of an arteriovenous malformation in a child. JAMA Dermatol 2019;155(2):256–7.

32. Derdeyn CP, Zipfel GJ, Albuquerque FC, et al. Management of brain arteriovenous malformations: a scientific statement for healthcare professionals from the American Heart Association/American Stroke Association. Stroke 2017;48(8):e200–24.

33. Brown RD Jr, Wiebers DO, Torner JC, et al. Frequency of intracranial hemorrhage as a presenting symptom and subtype analysis: a population-based study of intracranial vascular malformations in Olmsted Country, Minnesota. J Neurosurg 1996;85(1):29–32.

34. da Costa L, Wallace MC, Ter Brugge KG, et al. The natural history and predictive features of hemorrhage from brain arteriovenous malformations. Stroke 2009;40(1):100–5.

35. Ferrara AR. Brain arteriovenous malformations. Radiol Technol 2011;82(6):543mr–56mr.

36. Barbosa Do Prado L, Han C, Oh SP, et al. Recent advances in basic research for brain arteriovenous malformation. Int J Mol Sci 2019;20(21).

37. Maddy K, Chalamgari A, Ariwodo O, et al. An updated review on the genetics of arteriovenous malformations. Gene Protein Dis 2023;2(2).

38. Kritharis A, Al-Samkari H, Kuter DJ. Hereditary hemorrhagic telangiectasia: diagnosis and management from the hematologist's perspective. Haematologica 2018;103(9):1433–43.

39. Shovlin CL, Guttmacher AE, Buscarini E, et al. Diagnostic criteria for hereditary hemorrhagic telangiectasia (Rendu-Osler-Weber syndrome). Am J Med Genet 2000;91(1):66–7.

40. Faughnan ME, Mager JJ, Hetts SW, et al. Second international guidelines for the diagnosis and management of hereditary hemorrhagic telangiectasia. Ann Intern Med 2020;173(12):989–1001.

41. Rosenberg T, Fialla AD, Kjeldsen J, et al. Does severe bleeding in HHT patients respond to intravenous bevacizumab? Review of the literature and case series. Rhinology 2019;57(4):242–51.

42. Kjeldsen AD, Møller TR, Brusgaard K, et al. Clinical symptoms according to genotype amongst patients with hereditary haemorrhagic telangiectasia. J Intern Med 2005;258(4):349–55.

43. Donaldson JW, McKeever TM, Hall IP, et al. Complications and mortality in hereditary hemorrhagic telangiectasia: A population-based study. Neurology 2015;84(18):1886–93.

44. Kilian A, Latino GA, White AJ, et al. Genotype-phenotype correlations in children with HHT. J Clin Med 2020;9(9).

45. Tørring PM, Brusgaard K, Ousager LB, et al. National mutation study among Danish patients with hereditary haemorrhagic telangiectasia. Clin Genet 2014;86(2):123–33.

46. Balachandar S, Graves TJ, Shimonty A, et al. Identification and validation of a novel pathogenic variant in GDF2 (BMP9) responsible for hereditary hemorrhagic telangiectasia and pulmonary arteriovenous malformations. Am J Med Genet 2022;188(3):959–64.

47. Setty BA, Wusik K, Hammill AM. How we approach genetics in the diagnosis and management of vascular anomalies. Pediatr Blood Cancer 2022;69(Suppl 3):e29320.

48. Doh EJ, Ohn J, Kim MJ, et al. Prospective pilot study on combined use of pulsed dye laser and 1% topical rapamycin for treatment of nonfacial cutaneous capillary malformation. J Dermatol Treat 2017;28(7):672–7.

49. Hobayan CGP, Nourse EJ, Paradiso MM, et al. Delayed ulceration following combination pulse dye laser and topical sirolimus treatment for port wine birthmarks: A case series. Pediatr Dermatol 2023. https://doi.org/10.1111/pde.15409.

50. Sebold AJ, Day AM, Ewen J, et al. Sirolimus treatment in sturge-weber syndrome. Pediatr Neurol 2021;115:29–40.

Medical Therapeutics for the Treatment of Vascular Anomalies: Part 3

Kiersten Ricci, MD[a,b]

KEYWORDS

- Vascular anomaly • Vascular malformation • Sirolimus • Alpelisib • MEK inhibitor
- Angiogenesis inhibitor

KEY POINTS

- Most vascular anomalies are associated with mutations, most commonly somatic, disrupting tyrosine kinase receptor signaling through the PIK3/AKT and RAS/MAPK/MEK pathways.
- Molecularly targeted medical therapeutics are important treatment considerations in the interdisciplinary management of complicated vascular anomalies.
- Sirolimus, a potent mammalian target of rapamycin inhibitor, has been demonstrated to be a safe and efficacious treatment for complicated vascular anomalies in numerous studies.
- Currently, most nontargeted and molecularly targeted medications, other than alpelisib, are used off-label and on a compassionate basis for complicated management of vascular anomalies.
- Cost of genetic testing and procurement of molecularly targeted medications remain challenges in the care of complicated vascular anomalies.

INTRODUCTION

Optimal management of complex vascular anomalies aims to not only treat acute issues, such as infection or effusion, but also prevent potential future complications and improve physical functioning and quality of life. Historically, medical treatment for vascular anomalies focused on managing complications with supportive measures, such as pain control, antibiotics, dental hygiene, and compression garments. In addition to the creation of a formal classification system of vascular anomalies by the International Society for the Study of Vascular Anomalies, the serendipitous discovery of sirolimus, a mammalian target of rapamycin (mTOR) inhibitor, as an efficacious treatment for complicated vascular anomalies, boosted interest in the field, propelling clinical and basic science research, and began to shift the treatment paradigm.[1,2]

The study of the pathophysiology and molecular biology of vascular tumors and malformations has rapidly expanded. In the last decade, germline and somatic mutations in the endothelial receptor intracellular signaling pathways, phosphatidylinositol-4,5-bisphosphate 3-kinase (PIK3)/AKT and RAS/MAPK/MEK, have been identified in numerous vascular anomalies.[3–5] Overactivation of tyrosine kinase receptor signaling through the PIK3/AKT and RAS/MAPK/MEK pathways causes disruption of normal cellular activities, resulting in cellular proliferation, survival advantage, and angiogenesis, which is thought to be the mechanism driving the development and/or progression of vascular anomalies. Although optimal management of patients with complex vascular anomalies requires an interdisciplinary approach, these genomic discoveries have led to new therapeutic options and the increasing importance of the hematologist/oncologist within multidisciplinary vascular care teams. This article

[a] Division of Hematology, Cancer and Blood Diseases Institute, Hemangioma and Vascular Malformation Center, Cincinnati Children's Hospital Medical Center, 3333 Burnet Avenue, MLC 7015, Cincinnati, OH 45229, USA;
[b] University of Cincinnati College of Medicine, 231 Albert Sabin Way, Cincinnati, OH 45267-0558, USA
E-mail address: Kiersten.Ricci@cchmc.org

Oral Maxillofacial Surg Clin N Am 36 (2024) 125–136
https://doi.org/10.1016/j.coms.2023.09.013
1042-3699/24/© 2023 Elsevier Inc. All rights reserved.

discusses the use of molecularly targeted medications and anti-angiogenesis agents in the management of complicated vascular anomalies. **Table 1** lists the known associated genetic mutations for the various vascular anomaly phenotypes. **Fig. 1** illustrates the molecular targets of medications within the PIK3CA/AKT and RAS/MAPK/MEK pathways.

MAMMALIAN TARGET OF RAPAMYCIN INHIBITORS: SIROLIMUS/EVEROLIMUS

Sirolimus, also known as rapamycin, is a specific inhibitor of mTOR, a serine/threonine kinase in the PIK3/AKT pathway that regulates protein synthesis and cell growth through downstream signaling. Before use in vascular anomalies, sirolimus was used to treat individuals with tuberous sclerosis and lymphangioleiomyomatosis or LAM, conditions caused by TSC1 and TSC2 mutations that affect the PIK3/AKT pathway. Sirolimus was first used under compassionate-care protocol in a patient with kaposiform hemangioendothelioma, severe Kasabach-Merritt phenomenon (KMP), and multiorgan failure who was refractory to all previously known effective treatments, including corticosteroids, vincristine, cyclophosphamide, bevacizumab, and embolization. With sirolimus treatment, the patient had complete resolution of KMP as well as significant improvement in pain, lesion size, and functional abilities. Hammill and colleagues[2] also reported similar benefits in 4 other individuals with various complex vascular anomalies. Subsequently, a phase 2 clinical trial evaluating the safety of efficacy of sirolimus treatment in multiple complicated vascular anomalies revealed an overall response rate of 85% at 1 year of treatment with low toxicity.[6] Although radiologic disease improved in approximately half of the patients, most had improved clinical symptoms and/or quality of life. Given these encouraging

Table 1
Identified gene mutations by phenotype of associated vascular anomaly

Diagnosis/Phenotype	Genetic Mutations
Lymphatic malformation, sporadic	PIK3CA
Klippel-Trenaunay syndrome (capillary lymphatic venous malformation or capillary venous malformation with overgrowth of affected extremity)	PIK3CA
CLOVES syndrome	PIK3CA
Megalencephaly–capillary malformation (MCM) or Megalencephaly–capillary malformation–polymicrogyria syndrome (MCAP)	PIK3CA
Generalized lymphatic anomaly (GLA)	PIK3CA
Kaposiform lymphangiomatosis (KLA)	NRAS
Venous malformations, sporadic	PIK3CA, TIE2/TEK
Glomuvenous malformation	GLMN
Multiple cutaneous and mucosal venous malformation (VMCM)	TIE2/TEK
Blue rubber bleb nevus syndrome (BRBNS)	TIE2/TEK
Arteriovenous malformations, extracranial and sporadic	MAP2K1, KRAS, NRAS, BRAF
Arteriovenous malformation, intracranial and sporadic	KRAS, BRAF
Phosphatase and tensin homolog hamartoma	PTEN
Fibroadipose vascular anomaly	PIK3CA
Vein of Galen aneurysmal malformation, subtype of cerebral AVM	EPHB4
Capillary malformation–arteriovenous malformation type 1 (CM-AVM1)	RASA1
Capillary malformation–arteriovenous malformation type 2 (CM-AVM2)	EPHB4
Hereditary hemorrhagic telangiectasia syndrome (HHT)	ACVRL1, ENG, SMAD4, GDF2/BMP9
Capillary malformation, sporadic	GNAQ, GNA11
Sturge-Weber syndrome	GNAQ
Facial infiltrating lipomatosis	PIK3CA

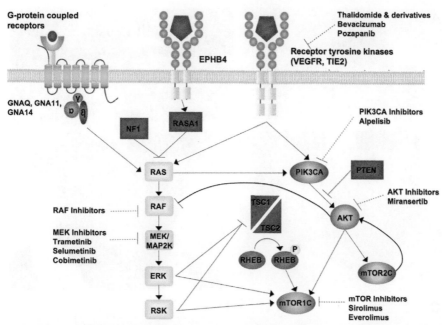

Fig. 1. Molecular targets of medications used in vascular anomalies within the PIK3CA/AKT and RAS/RAF/MEK pathways.

results, the use of sirolimus quickly expanded, proving efficacious in a wide variety of vascular tumors and malformations and demonstrating additional benefits when used in combination with surgery and interventional procedures.

As demonstrated in the phase 2 clinical trial, sirolimus is efficacious for the treatment of complex microcystic and macrocystic lymphatic malformations by inhibiting overactive PIK3/AKT signaling caused by the gain-of-function *PIK3CA* mutations in lymphatic malformations.[6] Numerous studies, along with case series and reports, have demonstrated similar benefits for lymphatic malformations and combined malformations with a lymphatic component.[7–16] Reduction of malformation size, cutaneous lymphatic lesions, malformation-associated infections, bleeding complications, and pain, along with improved quality of life, have all been reported with systemic sirolimus treatment. With minimal to no systemic absorption, topical sirolimus, now commercially available in the United States, has also shown benefit in treating cutaneous manifestations of lymphatic malformations by lessening the number or size of lymphatic vesicles as well as lymphatic leakage or bleeding from the skin.[17–20] From the author's clinical experience, some patients experience skin irritation or a sensation of burning, but alteration of the vehicle, that is, cream, ointment, or similar, can sometimes resolve this issue.

In the head and neck area, sirolimus has demonstrated importance in the multidisciplinary management of cervicofacial lymphatic malformation, as shown in **Fig. 2**. One case series of 8 infants with cervicofacial lymphatic malformations, refractory to sclerotherapy and/or surgery, responded positively to sirolimus therapy with modest to significant response with acceptable side effects.[21] Similarly, another case series of 19 patients with cervicofacial lymphatic malformations demonstrated similar efficacy with a reduction in malformation volume and improved or resolved mucosal vesicles while on sirolimus.[22] In a retrospective, multicenter review of 13 patients with an extensive lymphatic malformation of the head and neck region, who previously underwent placement of tracheostomy and subsequently received sirolimus treatment, Holm and colleagues[23] found that tracheostomy was able to be reversed in 62% of the patients with a median duration of 18 months of sirolimus treatment before tracheostomy removal. Sirolimus therapy has also shown significant improvements in macroglossia and oral/tongue bleeding secondary to lymphatic or venous lymphatic malformation.[24,25] Topical administration of sirolimus is currently being investigated for lingual microcystic lymphatic malformations (NCT04128722).

Sirolimus has also shown efficacy in the management of complex lymphatic anomalies, including generalized lymphatic anomalies (GLA), Gorham-Stout disease (GSD), and kaposiform lymphangiomatosis (KLA). In an analysis of 18 patients with GSD and GLA treated with systemic sirolimus,

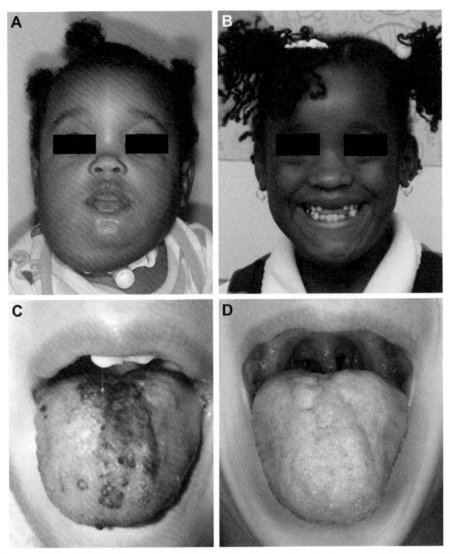

Fig. 2. Patients with lymphatic malformations (LM) involving the head and neck area on sirolimus treatment. (*A*) Infant with a large cervicofacial requiring tracheostomy, before sirolimus therapy. (*B*) On sirolimus therapy, the same child as in panel A, with a marked decrease of LM bulkiness and improved symmetry and tracheostomy no longer in place. (*C*) Older child with a microcystic LM involving the tongue with many cutaneous vesicles with frequent bleeding, before sirolimus. (*D*) On sirolimus therapy, same child as in panel C, with improved bulk and resolution of cutaneous vesicles and bleeding.

83% of the children and young adults had improvement in one or more aspects of their disease (quality of life, 78%; clinical status, 72%; imaging, 28%). Furthermore, bone disease did not progress, and pleural and pericardial effusions substantially improved in affected patients while on therapy.[9] Although bone disease did not progress in this study, the time to follow-up was relatively short (12–19 months), and patients with GSD, which has the propensity to affect the skull, vertebrae, and jaw, only constituted 28% of the small cohort. Sirolimus has also shown benefit as monotherapy and in combined regimens with steroids and

vincristine for the treatment of KLA by improving coagulopathy, pleural and pericardial effusions, ascites, respiratory issues, and bleeding complications.[11,26–30] Although KLA is now known to be associated with an *NRAS* mutation, the beneficial effect of sirolimus in some patients with this rare disease is presumably because of substantial cross talk between the PI3K/AKT and RAS/MAPK/MEK pathways at different stages of signal propagation.

In some individuals with venous malformations or with combined malformations with a venous component, sirolimus has also shown benefits.

Pure venous malformations were excluded from the original phase 2 clinical trial, but combined malformations with a venous component were included. One study combining the phase 2 results with a retrospective trial of patients with capillary lymphatic venous malformation demonstrated that disease-related bleeding improved in all affected patients while on therapy. A significant reduction in recurrent thrombophlebitis/phlebolithiasis was also reported.[10] Another case series of 19 individuals, including children and adults, with slow-flow vascular malformations treated with sirolimus showed similar improvement in coagulopathy.[31] A case series of 6 individuals with pure venous malformations who were no longer responsive to standard therapies reported improvement in bleeding episodes, intensity or frequency of pain, volume of affected body part or parts, and functional limitations.[32] Improvement has been more evident clinically versus that published. For example, the author reports one case of a patient with significant macroglossia, secondary to presumed venous and lymphatic disease. Upon treatment with low-dose sirolimus since infancy, the venous and lymphatic malformation components substantially lessened clinically and radiologically over time (**Fig. 3**). Multiple other case reports and small case series have also reported benefits for venous malformations.[14,33,34] In Europe, a prospective multicenter phase 3 trial (NCT02638389) is investigating the use of sirolimus in venous malformations and lymphatic malformations in which conventional therapies, such as surgery or sclerotherapy, have been ineffective or not recommended owing to high-risk important complications. Most venous malformations are associated with *PIK3CA* or *TIE2/TEK* mutations, and therefore, are more likely to respond to sirolimus therapy. Differences in the vessel endothelium type and exposure to blood and its components in comparison to lymphatic fluid could potentially account for the different responses to sirolimus in venous versus lymphatic malformations.

Efficacy data of sirolimus in capillary malformations, arteriovenous malformations (AVM), and other high-flow combined lesions are limited. Phosphatase and tensin homolog hamartoma tumor syndrome (PTHS) is characterized by the formation of recurrent benign tumors of soft tissue that may contain fast-flow vascular anomalies. Sirolimus has been beneficial in improving pain and function in some patients with PTHS.[35,36] One retrospective study of 9 patients with high-flow lesions (8 AVM, 1 arteriovenous fistula) reported improvement in all but one patient with a reduction in bleeding episodes, decreased size

of the lesion, and/or stabilization over time.[37] However, other case series reported a poor efficacy of sirolimus in patients with extracranial AVM.[38,39] One small prospective study investigated the use of oral sirolimus in children with Sturge-Weber syndrome and suggested that sirolimus may be beneficial for cognitive impairments, such as in those with impaired processing speed or a history of strokelike episodes.[40] Systemic and topical sirolimus have not demonstrated any benefits for capillary malformations or the capillary components of combined malformations.[6,41,42] In fact, combined use of topical sirolimus and pulsed dye laser for treatment of capillary malformation (CM) may result in increased complications, such as delayed ulceration and increased systemic absorption.[42]

Sirolimus is taken orally once or twice a day as a pill or liquid suspension. In the phase 2 clinical trial, sirolimus was started at 0.8 mg/m^2 per dosage every 12 hours and titrated to maintain a serum trough level of 10 to 15 ng/mL. Since the trial, lower target trough levels have been shown to be effective in patients with vascular anomalies. As a result, many clinicians now titrate the sirolimus dose to achieve the desired benefit without significant adverse effects. Generally, low-/intermediate-dose sirolimus (levels <8 ng/mL) is typically used for symptomatic relief, whereas high-dose sirolimus (levels >8 ng/mL) is reserved for patients with severe coagulopathy, multiorgan failure, and/or life-threatening lesions. Clearance of sirolimus in neonates and young children differs from that in older children and adults. Suggested sirolimus starting doses for newborns and young children have recently been described based on pharmacokinetics.[43] The most common side effects are mouth sores, gastrointestinal (GI) upset, headaches, bone marrow suppression, and metabolic/laboratory abnormalities. While the patient is on therapy, regular physical examinations and laboratory bloodwork are required to guarantee adequate drug levels and to monitor for toxicities. *Pneumocystis jiroveci* pneumonia prophylaxis is generally recommended given immunosuppressive effects, particularly in neonates. Although each patient's response time differs, maximal benefit typically does not occur until months after achieving adequate dosing. Treatment duration must be established on an individual basis.

Everolimus has a similar molecular mechanism to sirolimus, albeit different, and thus, has a different clinical profile. Comparative pharmacokinetics suggest that everolimus is more readily absorbed and has higher oral bioavailability, quicker steady-state blood concentration after initiation, and faster elimination after discontinuation in comparison to

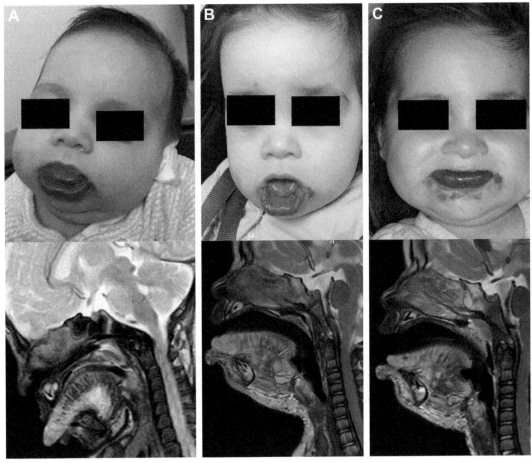

Fig. 3. Correlating MRI of a child with a facial venous lymphatic malformation treated with sirolimus alone. (*A*) Infant at the age of ~2 months, around the time of oral sirolimus initiation. On examination, the baby had significant macroglossia with the inability to close the mouth. MRI shows that the tongue is significantly enlarged, filling the oral cavity and oropharynx, and increased T2 signal throughout from the base to the tip. Of note, this child also has other areas of involvement not represented in these images. (*B*) The same child, on low-dose sirolimus therapy, at approximately 1 year of age with clinical improvement in the bulkiness of her malformation within the tongue as well as the soft tissue of her face. MRI demonstrates continued T2 enhancement of the tongue but overall is reduced with less filling of the oral cavity and oropharynx. (*C*) Same individual after ~2 years of sirolimus therapy. Clinically, the patient has mild macroglossia with ability to hold in/close the mouth in addition to normal speech development for age. MRI demonstrates further reduction in bulk of the tongue. Of note, there is a small phlebolith near the tip of the tongue that was asymptomatic.

sirolimus.[44] Despite these potentially advantageous pharmacokinetic differences, data are very limited on the use of everolimus in the treatment of vascular anomalies. However, everolimus is a treatment consideration in those with intolerable side effects from sirolimus or in those without access to sirolimus.

MIRANSERTIB

AKT is a critical component of the cellular PIK3CA-AKT-mTOR pathway, and thus, has been a potential molecular target for the treatment of individuals with vascular malformations and associated syndromes within this pathway, but efficacy data remain limited. Miransertib is an oral pan-AKT inhibitor that inhibits both active and inactive forms of AKT. Miransertib was initially developed for cancer therapeutics but is now being trialed for PIK3CA-related overgrowth spectrum (PROS) and Proteus syndrome, an overgrowth syndrome caused by somatic mutation of AKT1. In both in vitro and in vivo experiments, the drug demonstrated antiproliferative activity in cells derived from patients with PROS and Proteus syndrome.[45,46] In preliminary results of an open-label, phase 1/2 study of MOSAIC (miransertib in patients with PROS and Proteus Syndrome), most patients experienced improvement in disease-related symptoms and performance status as measured by the Karnofsky/Lansky scale, and most demonstrated improvement or no disease progression extending beyond 1 year on treatment. Preliminary results also reported that miransertib had a manageable safety profile in patients as young as 2 years old, with mostly grade 1 or 2 adverse events.[47,48] On a compassionate-use basis, Forde and colleagues[49] treated 2 pediatric patients, one with CLOVES and one with facial infiltrating lipomatosis and hemimegaloencephaly, with miransertib and noted clinical response in the patient with CLOVES and improvement in key qualitative outcomes in the other.

ALPELISIB

Alpelisib (BYL719) is an oral, selective alpha-specific PI3K inhibitor that directly targets PIK3CA activating mutations, and thus, has been a very attractive therapeutic target for lymphatic and venous malformations as well as PROS, which includes Klippel-Trenaunay syndrome and CLOVES syndrome. Alpelisib has been used for various tumors with PIK3 gain-of-function mutations, with most of its use in the treatment of breast cancer. In individuals with breast cancer, alpelisib has been generally well tolerated with the most common side effects being hyperglycemia and mouth sores.

In the initial studies of alpelisib in vascular anomalies, Venot and colleagues[50] developed a mouse model that mimicked PROS in humans and demonstrated that alpelisib (BYL719) not only increased survival (in comparison to mice given placebo) but also reduced disease when given to phenotypic/affected mice. Furthermore, the group also found that, in fibroblasts from the PROS mice, alpelisib (BYL719) inhibited AKT more efficiently than sirolimus, potentially because of more mTORC2 inhibition. Under compassionate-care protocols, Venot and colleagues[50] then administered alpelisib (BYL719) to 2 patients with severe clinical manifestations of PROS/CLOVES and confirmed somatic PIK3CA mutations. Both individuals experienced significant vascular tumor shrinkage and improved symptoms by 12 to 18 months on drug treatment. Subsequently, the group expanded use of BYL719 (alpelisib) to 17 additional individuals with PROS (6 CLOVES, 2 megalencephaly capillary malformation, 3 localized overgrowth, and 3 with abdominal or chest tumors) and gain-of-function PIK3CA mutations, and all were reported to have clinical improvement and radiologic response. Venot and colleagues[50] reported that alpelisib was well tolerated and that hyperglycemia was adequately controlled with dietary changes. Although these results are very encouraging, the study was not prospective and was limited to a small number of patients with severe disease only.

Additional case reports and small case series have since been published reporting the benefits of alpelisib in PROS. Morin and colleagues[51] reported the safety and efficacy of alpelisib 25 mg once daily in 2 young children (8 months of age, and 9 months of age) with PROS. One of the children had hemimegaloencephaly with increased volume of the right hemisphere with associated infantile spasms and seizure activity, and upon starting alpelisib, epilepsy improved clinically and on electroencephalogram. Alpelisib was also reported to reduce mesenteric lymphatic disease and improve pain, reducing opioid use by 50%, in an adult with PROS with capillary lymphatic venous malformation.[52] Another group reported benefit of alpelisib in a young girl with CLOVES syndrome and combined vascular malformation involving her genitalia who suffered from abnormal vaginal bleeding requiring blood transfusion despite sirolimus treatment. On alpelisib, the vaginal bleeding resolved, and tissue bulkiness decreased, allowing for surgical debulking and reconstruction.[53] Multiple other case reports have also emerged reporting clinical improvements in patients with PROS with or without vascular malformations treated with alpelisib after sirolimus was deemed inadequate.[54,55] In patients with megalencephaly-capillary malformation, the use of alpelisib to control hypoglycemic episodes and/or seizures has been suggested but not prospectively studied to date.

In the United States, the retrospective chart review on patients with PROS above the age of 2 years with severe disease, the EPIK-P1 study (NCT04285723), also demonstrated the clinical efficacy of alpelisib in this patient population. Of the 32 patients with complete data, 37.5% had at least a 20% reduction in tumor size, and most had clinical improvements. The phase 2 multicenter clinical trial (EPIK-P2) with an upfront 16-week, randomized, double-blind, placebo-controlled period, to assess the efficacy, safety, and pharmacokinetics of alpelisib in pediatric and adult participants with PROS is currently ongoing (NCT04589650). Alpelisib for the treatment of other PIK3CA-related malformations is planned in upcoming trials. Specific PIK3CA inhibition is an exciting new therapeutic target for lymphatic malformations because most are associated with PIK3CA activating mutations.

MEK INHIBITORS

Several vascular anomalies, including extracranial AVM, capillary malformation–arteriovenous malformation (CM-AVM), and KLA, carry mutations that result in constitutive activation of the RAS/MAPK/MEK signaling pathway, conferring a significant selective growth advantage. Currently, data are limited on the use of MEK inhibitors, such as trametinib, selumetinib, and cobimetinib, in vascular anomalies that are associated with mutations of the RAS/MAPK/MEK pathway. However, clinical use is increasing, particularly in those with inadequate response to conventional treatments, in addition to increased knowledge of genotype/phenotype correlations.

Published data on MEK inhibition in vascular anomalies remain limited. In one patient with a lymphatic conduction disorder and associated RAF mutation, Li and colleagues[56] reported that MEK inhibition resulted in remodeling of the patient's lymphatic system and symptom resolution. Chowers and colleagues[57] reported that a patient with KLA, who had received steroids, propranolol, diuretics, thalidomide, and sirolimus alone or in combination, was treated with trametinib, and subsequently, had improvement in coagulopathy, lung function and oxygen support, and quality of life. Similarly, Foster and colleagues[58] described a patient with KLA, previously treated with steroids, vincristine, interferon, and sirolimus, who developed worsening pulmonary disease; with trametinib treatment, the patient experienced improvement in respiratory symptoms and exercise tolerance, as well as resolution of pleural effusions and pulmonary edema. Trametinib therapy was also shown to improve bleeding and the appearance of a complex MAP2K1-associated AVM of the ear and neck in a pediatric patient.[59] Nicholson and colleagues[60] used trametinib therapy in an adolescent with CM-AVM2 with innumerable arteriovenous shunts and dominant nidus of the lower extremity, along with early high-output cardiac failure, and reported improvement of shunting by cardiac catheterization at 10 months on therapy. In the United States, 2 trials investigating the use of MEK inhibitors in extracranial AVMs are ongoing (NCT04258046, NCT05125471). Given the rarity of CM-AVM and KLA, prospective studies on treatment with MEK inhibitors are likely infeasible. Although studies are limited, systemic MEK inhibition for vascular lesions needs to be considered within the multidisciplinary treatment plan, as diseases associated with RAS pathway mutations are often progressive.

ANTIANGIOGENESIS AGENTS

After years of nonuse due to teratogenicity, oral thalidomide was discovered to have antiangiogenic effects in 1994.[61] One randomized controlled trial reported that thalidomide effectively treated GI angiodysplasia-associated bleeding, finding that individuals taking thalidomide as opposed to control with oral iron had fewer hospitalizations, bleeding episodes, and blood transfusion requirements.[62] In individuals with hereditary hemorrhagic telangiectasia syndrome (HHT), thalidomide has been shown to decrease the frequency and severity of nosebleeds, raise hemoglobin levels, and lessen transfusion requirements.[63–66] Not only is its use restricted because of teratogenicity but thalidomide is also sedating and can cause peripheral neuropathy with long-term usage. Lenalidomide and pomalidomide are oral thalidomide derivatives that have antiangiogenic effects but less reported sedating effects and risk for peripheral neuropathy. The phase 2 placebo-controlled double-blind study of pomalidomide in patients with HHT is ongoing (NCT03910244).

Pazopanib, an oral multitarget VEGF receptor tyrosine kinase inhibitor, recently demonstrated benefit in the treatment of individuals with HHT. One observational analysis of 13 patients with severe HHT-associated bleeding and red cell transfusion-dependent anemia reported an excellent response with low-dose oral pazopanib. On pazopanib therapy, all patients achieved transfusion independence. After 3 months of treatment, red blood cell transfusions decreased by 93%, and intravenous iron infusions reduced by 92%. Pazopanib was reported to be well tolerated with the most common side effects being hypertension, lymphocytopenia, and fatigue.[67] Additional studies are needed to determine the effectiveness of pazopanib in HHT and similar vascular conditions associated with bleeding complications.

Bevacizumab is a recombinant humanized monoclonal antibody, administered intravenously, that binds to VEGF receptors on endothelial cells and acts as a competitive antagonist. Bevacizumab has recently emerged as a targeted antiangiogenic therapy for HHT-associated bleeding. The multicenter observational InHIBIT-Bleed study of 238 patients with HHT receiving bevacizumab demonstrated improvements in mean hemoglobin and a reduction in the epistaxis severity score at 1 year on treatment. Remarkedly, the study also found that on 6 months of therapy, red blood cell transfusion declined by 82% and iron infusions decreased by 70%.[68] One study of 25 patients with HHT associated with severe hepatic vascular malformations and high cardiac output found that bevacizumab decreased cardiac output and reduced the duration and number of episodes of epistaxis.[69] In the InHIBIT-Bleed study, systemic bevacizumab was administered as a series of 4 to 6 induction infusions dosed at 5 mg/kg every 2 weeks, followed by maintenance treatment in individuals demonstrating response.[68]

TREATMENT CHALLENGES

The prevalence of vascular anomalies is estimated at 5%, whereas the prevalence of vascular malformations is 1.5% of the general population. Thus, vascular anomalies are not rare, and this approximation is grossly underrated. Presumed rarity is due to widespread medical provider unfamiliarity of these diseases, along with a scarcity of multidisciplinary centers caring for these vascular anomalies, and in particular, those caring for adults. Although the importance of phenotype and genotype correlation has become increasingly important in the treatment of patients with complex vascular anomalies, somatic genetic testing of tissue remains very difficult to obtain without patients taking on a substantial financial burden. In addition, genetic testing of vascular anomalies remains difficult because of the low-allele frequency of mutation needed for detection. Without confirmation of the genetic mutation within the malformation, many patients who would benefit from disease-modifying medications currently are unable to obtain targeted therapy because of medical coverage issues.

SUMMARY

Clinical and scientific research, technological advances, and genomic discoveries have improved the understanding of the clinical behavior, pathologic condition, and molecular biology of vascular anomalies. Germline and somatic mutations associated with vascular anomalies result in overactivation of the PIK3/AKT and/or RAS/MAPK/MEK intracellular signaling pathway. Multiple inhibitors of these pathways and anti-angiogenesis agents, approved for use in the treatment of malignancies, have been used mostly off-label and demonstrated safety and effectiveness in complicated vascular anomalies and associated syndromes. Molecularly targeted therapies should be considered a primary treatment option for complex vascular anomalies as well as an adjunct to surgical interventions.

CLINICS CARE POINTS

- Systemic sirolimus treatment is safe and has a tolerable side effect profile for individuals of all ages with vascular anomalies.
- Initial sirolimus dosing in neonates and infants with vascular anomalies was determined by pharmacokinetic studies.
- Alpelisib is FDA-approved for the treatment of pediatric (2 years and older) and adult

patients with severe manifestations of PIK3CA-related overgrowth spectrum.
- Somatic genetic testing of vascular anomalies remains challenging to obtain and is often costly.

DISCLOSURE

The author declares no conflicts of interest related to this manuscript.

REFERENCES

1. ISSVA Classification of vascular anomalies 2018, International Society for the Study of Vascular Anomalies. Available at "issva.org/classification" Accessed July 22, 2023. . https://www.issva.org/UserFiles/file/ISSVA-Classification-2018.pdf. Accessed July 18, 2023.
2. Hammill AM, Wentzel M, Gupta A, et al. Sirolimus for the treatment of complicated vascular anomalies in children. Pediatr Blood Cancer 2011;57(6): 1018–24.
3. Greene AK, Goss JA. Vascular Anomalies: From a Clinicohistologic to a Genetic Framework. Plast Reconstr Surg 2018;141(5):709e–17e.
4. Wassef M, Blei F, Adams D, et al. Vascular Anomalies Classification: Recommendations From the International Society for the Study of Vascular Anomalies. Pediatrics 2015;136(1):e203–14.
5. Queisser A, Seront E, Boon LM, et al. Genetic Basis and Therapies for Vascular Anomalies. Circ Res 2021;129(1):155–73.
6. Adams DM, Trenor CC 3rd, Hammill AM, et al. Efficacy and Safety of Sirolimus in the Treatment of Complicated Vascular Anomalies. Pediatrics 2016; 137(2):e20153257.
7. Alba-Linero C, García-Lorente M, Rachwani-Anil R, et al. Treatment of orbital lymphatic malformation with oral sirolimus: a case report. Arq Bras Oftalmol 2022;S0004. 27492022005006218.
8. Teng JMC, Hammill A, Martini J, et al. Sirolimus in the Treatment of Microcystic Lymphatic Malformations: A Systematic Review. Lymphat Res Biol 2023;21(2): 101–10.
9. Ricci KW, Hammill AM, Mobberley-Schuman P, et al. Efficacy of systemic sirolimus in the treatment of generalized lymphatic anomaly and Gorham-Stout disease. Pediatr Blood Cancer 2019;66(5):e27614.
10. Engel ER, Hammill A, Adams D, et al. Response to sirolimus in capillary lymphatic venous malformations and associated syndromes: Impact on symptomatology, quality of life, and radiographic response. Pediatr Blood Cancer 2023;70(4):e30215.
11. Ozeki M, Nozawa A, Yasue S, et al. The impact of sirolimus therapy on lesion size, clinical symptoms,

and quality of life of patients with lymphatic anomalies. Orphanet J Rare Dis 2019;14(1):141.

12. Laforgia N, Schettini F, De Mattia D, et al. Lymphatic Malformation in Newborns as the First Sign of Diffuse Lymphangiomatosis: Successful Treatment with Sirolimus. Neonatology 2016;109(1):52–5.

13. Curry S, Logeman A, Jones D. Sirolimus: A Successful Medical Treatment for Head and Neck Lymphatic Malformations. Case Rep Otolaryngol 2019;2019: 2076798.

14. Harbers VEM, Rongen G, van der Vleuten CJM, et al. Patients with Congenital Low-Flow Vascular Malformation Treated with Low Dose Sirolimus. Adv Ther 2021;38(6):3465–82.

15. Tian R, Liang Y, Zhang W, et al. Effectiveness of sirolimus in the treatment of complex lymphatic malformations: Single center report of 56 cases. J Pediatr Surg 2020;55(11):2454–8.

16. Alemi AS, Rosbe KW, Chan DK, et al. Airway response to sirolimus therapy for the treatment of complex pediatric lymphatic malformations. Int J Pediatr Otorhinolaryngol 2015;79(12):2466–9.

17. Badia P, Ricci K, Gurria JP, et al. Topical sirolimus for the treatment of cutaneous manifestations of vascular anomalies: A case series. Pediatr Blood Cancer 2020;67(4):e28088.

18. Çalışkan E, Altunel CT, Özkan CK, et al. A case of microcystic lymphatic malformation successfully treated with topical sirolimus. Dermatol Ther 2018; 31(5):e12673.

19. Le Sage S, David M, Dubois J, et al. Efficacy and absorption of topical sirolimus for the treatment of vascular anomalies in children: A case series. Pediatr Dermatol 2018;35(4):472–7.

20. García-Montero P, Del Boz J, Baselga-Torres E, et al. Use of topical rapamycin in the treatment of superficial lymphatic malformations. J Am Acad Dermatol 2019;80(2):508–15.

21. Wu C, Song D, Guo L, et al. Refractory Head and Neck Lymphatic Malformation in Infants Treated With Sirolimus: A Case Series. Front Oncol 2021; 11:616702.

22. Strychowsky JE, Rahbar R, O'Hare MJ, et al. Sirolimus as treatment for 19 patients with refractory cervicofacial lymphatic malformation. Laryngoscope 2018;128(1):269–76.

23. Holm A, Te Loo M, Schultze Kool L, et al. Efficacy of Sirolimus in Patients Requiring Tracheostomy for Life-Threatening Lymphatic Malformation of the Head and Neck: A Report From the European Reference Network. Frontiers in pediatrics 2021;9:697960.

24. Yesil S, Bozkurt C, Tanyildiz HG, et al. Successful Treatment of Macroglossia Due to Lymphatic Malformation With Sirolimus. Ann Otol Rhinol Laryngol 2015;124(10):820–3.

25. Ghariani Fetoui N, Boussofara L, Gammoudi R, et al. Efficacy of sirolimus in the treatment of microcystic lymphatic malformation of the tongue. J Eur Acad Dermatol Venereol 2019;33(9):e336–7.

26. Zhou J, Yang K, Chen S, et al. Sirolimus in the treatment of kaposiform lymphangiomatosis. Orphanet J Rare Dis 2021;16(1):260.

27. Triana P, Dore M, Cerezo VN, et al. Sirolimus in the Treatment of Vascular Anomalies. Eur J Pediatr Surg 2017;27(1):86–90.

28. Wang Z, Li K, Yao W, et al. Successful treatment of kaposiform lymphangiomatosis with sirolimus. Pediatr Blood Cancer 2015;62(7):1291–3.

29. Crane J, Manfredo J, Boscolo E, et al. Kaposiform lymphangiomatosis treated with multimodal therapy improves coagulopathy and reduces blood angiopoietin-2 levels. Pediatr Blood Cancer 2020; 67(9):e28529.

30. Fernandes VM, Fargo JH, Saini S, et al. Kaposiform lymphangiomatosis: unifying features of a heterogeneous disorder. Pediatr Blood Cancer 2015;62(5): 901–4.

31. Hammer J, Seront E, Duez S, et al. Sirolimus is efficacious in treatment for extensive and/or complex slow-flow vascular malformations: a monocentric prospective phase II study. Orphanet J Rare Dis 2018;13(1):191.

32. Boscolo E, Limaye N, Huang L, et al. Rapamycin improves TIE2-mutated venous malformation in murine model and human subjects. J Clin Invest 2015; 125(9):3491–504.

33. Abdelbaky MA, Ragab IA, AbouZeid AA, et al. Sirolimus: A Rescue Drug to Control Complications of Extensive Venous Malformation. Eur J Pediatr Surg Rep 2020;8(1):e90–4.

34. Goldenberg DC, Carvas M, Adams D, et al. Successful Treatment of a Complex Vascular Malformation With Sirolimus and Surgical Resection. J Pediatr Hematol Oncol 2017;39(4):e191–5.

35. Iacobas I, Burrows PE, Adams DM, et al. Oral rapamycin in the treatment of patients with hamartoma syndromes and PTEN mutation. Pediatr Blood Cancer 2011;57(2):321–3.

36. Pimpalwar S, Yoo R, Chau A, et al. Temporal Evolution and Management of Fast Flow Vascular Anomalies in PTEN Hamartoma Tumor Syndrome. Int J Angiol 2018;27(3):158–64.

37. Durán-Romero AJ, Hernández-Rodríguez JC, Ortiz-Álvarez J, et al. Efficacy and safety of oral sirolimus for high-flow vascular malformations in real clinical practice. Clin Exp Dermatol 2022;47(1):57–62.

38. Gabeff R, Boccara O, Soupre V, et al. Efficacy and Tolerance of Sirolimus (Rapamycin) for Extracranial Arteriovenous Malformations in Children and Adults. Acta Derm Venereol 2019;99(12):1105–9.

39. Freixo C, Ferreira V, Martins J, et al. Efficacy and safety of sirolimus in the treatment of vascular anomalies: A systematic review. J Vasc Surg 2020;71(1): 318–27.

40. Sebold AJ, Day AM, Ewen J, et al. Sirolimus treatment in Sturge-Weber syndrome. Pediatr Neurol 2021;115:29–40.

41. Doh EJ, Ohn J, Kim MJ, et al. Prospective pilot study on combined use of pulsed dye laser and 1% topical rapamycin for treatment of nonfacial cutaneous capillary malformation. J Dermatol Treat 2017;28(7):672–7.

42. Hobayan CGP, Nourse EJ, Paradiso MM, Fernandez Faith E. Delayed ulceration following combination pulse dye laser and topical sirolimus treatment for port wine birthmarks: A case series. Pediatr Dermatol 2023. https://doi.org/10.1111/pde.15409.

43. Mizuno T, Fukuda T, Emoto C, et al. Developmental pharmacokinetics of sirolimus: Implications for precision dosing in neonates and infants with complicated vascular anomalies. Pediatr Blood Cancer 2017;64(8). https://doi.org/10.1002/pbc.26470.

44. MacKeigan JP, Krueger DA. Differentiating the mTOR inhibitors everolimus and sirolimus in the treatment of tuberous sclerosis complex. Neuro Oncol 2015;17(12):1550–9.

45. Yu Y, Savage RE, Eathiraj S, et al. Targeting AKT1-E17K and the PI3K/AKT Pathway with an Allosteric AKT Inhibitor, ARQ 092. PLoS One 2015;10(10): e0140479.

46. Lindhurst MJ, Yourick MR, Yu Y, et al. Repression of AKT signaling by ARQ 092 in cells and tissues from patients with Proteus syndrome. Sci Rep 2015;5: 17162.

47. Zampino G LC, Buonuomo PS, Rana I, Onesimo R, Macchiaiolo M, et al. . An open-label, phase 1/2 study of miransertib (ARQ 092), an oral pan-AKT inhibitor, in patients (pts) with PIK3CA-related Overgrowth Spectrum (PROS) and Proteus Syndrome (PS): study design and preliminary results (NCT03094832). . Paper presented at: European Society of Human Genetics Conference; June 15-18, 2019; Gothenburg, Sweden.

48. Canaud G, Hammill AM, Adams D, et al. A review of mechanisms of disease across PIK3CA-related disorders with vascular manifestations. Orphanet J Rare Dis 2021;16(1):306.

49. Forde K, Resta N, Ranieri C, et al. Clinical experience with the AKT1 inhibitor miransertib in two children with PIK3CA-related overgrowth syndrome. Orphanet J Rare Dis 2021;16(1):109.

50. Venot Q, Blanc T, Rabia SH, et al. Targeted therapy in patients with PIK3CA-related overgrowth syndrome. Nature 2018;558(7711):540–6.

51. Morin G, Degrugillier-Chopinet C, Vincent M, et al. Treatment of two infants with PIK3CA-related overgrowth spectrum by alpelisib. J Exp Med 2022; 219(3):e20212148.

52. Garneau AP, Haydock L, Tremblay LE, et al. Somatic non-cancerous PIK3CA-related overgrowth syndrome treated with alpelisib in North America. J Mol Med (Berl) 2021;99(3):311–3.

53. López Gutiérrez JC, Lizarraga R, Delgado C, et al. Alpelisib Treatment for Genital Vascular Malformation in a Patient with Congenital Lipomatous Overgrowth, Vascular Malformations, Epidermal Nevi, and Spinal/Skeletal Anomalies and/or Scoliosis (CLOVES) Syndrome. J Pediatr Adolesc Gynecol 2019;32(6):648–50.

54. Garreta Fontelles G, Pardo Pastor J, Grande Moreillo C. Alpelisib to treat CLOVES syndrome, a member of the PIK3CA-related overgrowth syndrome spectrum. Br J Clin Pharmacol 2022;88(8): 3891–5.

55. Pagliazzi A, Oranges T, Traficante G, et al. PIK3CA-Related Overgrowth Spectrum From Diagnosis to Targeted Therapy: A Case of CLOVES Syndrome Treated With Alpelisib. Frontiers in pediatrics 2021; 9:732836.

56. Li D, March ME, Gutierrez-Uzquiza A, et al. ARAF recurrent mutation causes central conducting lymphatic anomaly treatable with a MEK inhibitor. Nat Med 2019;25(7):1116–22.

57. Chowers G, Abebe-Campino G, Golan H, et al. Treatment of severe Kaposiform lymphangiomatosis positive for NRAS mutation by MEK inhibition. Pediatr Res 2022. https://doi.org/10.1038/s41390-022-01986-06-0. https://doi.org/10.1038/s41390-022-0198.

58. Foster JB, Li D, March ME, et al. Kaposiform lymphangiomatosis effectively treated with MEK inhibition. EMBO Mol Med 2020;12(10):e12324.

59. Al-Samkari H, Eng W. A precision medicine approach to hereditary hemorrhagic telangiectasia and complex vascular anomalies. J Thromb Haemost 2022;20(5):1077–88.

60. Nicholson CL, Flanagan S, Murati M, et al. Successful management of an arteriovenous malformation with trametinib in a patient with capillary-malformation arteriovenous malformation syndrome and cardiac compromise. Pediatr Dermatol 2022;39(2):316–9.

61. D'Amato RJ, Loughnan MS, Flynn E, et al. Thalidomide is an inhibitor of angiogenesis. Proc Natl Acad Sci U S A 1994;91(9):4082–5.

62. Ge ZZ, Chen HM, Gao YJ, et al. Efficacy of thalidomide for refractory gastrointestinal bleeding from vascular malformation. Gastroenterology 2011; 141(5):1629–37. e1621-1624.

63. Harrison L, Kundra A, Jervis P. The use of thalidomide therapy for refractory epistaxis in hereditary haemorrhagic telangiectasia: systematic review. J Laryngol Otol 2018;132(10):866–71.

64. Baysal M, Ümit EG, Kırkızlar HO, et al. Thalidomide for the Management of Bleeding Episodes in Patients with Hereditary Hemorrhagic Telangiectasia: Effects on Epistaxis Severity Score and Quality of Life. Turk J Haematol 2019;36(1):43–7.

65. Franchini M, Lippi G. Thalidomide for hereditary haemorrhagic telangiectasia. Lancet Haematol 2015;2(11):e457–8.

66. Invernizzi R, Quaglia F, Klersy C, et al. Efficacy and safety of thalidomide for the treatment of severe recurrent epistaxis in hereditary haemorrhagic telangiectasia: results of a non-randomised, single-centre, phase 2 study. Lancet Haematol 2015;2(11):e465–73.

67. Parambil JG, Gossage JR, McCrae KR, et al. Pazopanib for severe bleeding and transfusion-dependent anemia in hereditary hemorrhagic telangiectasia. Angiogenesis 2022;25(1):87–97.

68. Al-Samkari H, Kasthuri RS, Parambil JG, et al. An international, multicenter study of intravenous bevacizumab for bleeding in hereditary hemorrhagic telangiectasia: the InHIBIT-Bleed study. Haematologica 2021;106(8):2161–9.

69. Dupuis-Girod S, Ginon I, Saurin JC, et al. Bevacizumab in patients with hereditary hemorrhagic telangiectasia and severe hepatic vascular malformations and high cardiac output. JAMA 2012;307(9):948–55.

Moving?

Make sure your subscription moves with you!

To notify us of your new address, find your **Clinics Account Number** (located on your mailing label above your name), and contact customer service at:

Email: **journalscustomerservice-usa@elsevier.com**

800-654-2452 (subscribers in the U.S. & Canada)
314-447-8871 (subscribers outside of the U.S. & Canada)

Fax number: 314-447-8029

Elsevier Health Sciences Division
Subscription Customer Service
3251 Riverport Lane
Maryland Heights, MO 63043

ELSEVIER

Printed and bound by CPI Group (UK) Ltd, Croydon, CR0 4YY

08/05/2025

01864747-0011